"An important and fascinating journey to answer one of life's most mysterious questions—why we age and how to do it well."

—David A. Kessler, MD, former commissioner, U.S. Food and Drug Administration; author, *The End of Overeating*

"A comprehensive look at what pertains to all of us—the science behind healthy aging."

—Stephanie Lederman, executive director, American Federation for Aging Research

"This book will likely inspire people from all over the world to take control of their health and the way they age."

—Bahram H. Arjmandi, PhD, RD; chair, Department of Nutrition, Food, and Exercise Sciences; director, Center for Advancing Exercise and Nutrition Research on Aging, Florida State University

"Margaret Pressler has found a fountain of youth in her own backyard. By describing the simple ways that her husband has slowed the usual effects of aging, she provides an easy roadmap that readers can follow—focusing on the basics of nutrition, exercise, sleep, and good health. Can there be anyone who wouldn't want to join the Presslers and 'Cheat the Clock'?"

—David Ignatius, columnist, *The Washington Post*

cheat

THE

clock

How New Science Can Help You
Look and Feel Younger

cheat
THE
clock

Margaret Webb Pressler
of *The Washington Post*

ALPHA

A member of Penguin Group (USA) Inc.

For Eleanor, Phoebe, and William. The best.

ALPHA BOOKS

Note: This publication contains the opinions and ideas of its author. It is intended to provide helpful and informative material on the subject matter covered. It is sold with the understanding that the author and publisher are not engaged in rendering professional services in the book. If the reader requires personal assistance or advice, a competent professional should be consulted.

The author and publisher specifically disclaim any responsibility for any liability, loss, or risk, personal or otherwise, which is incurred as a consequence, directly or indirectly, of the use and application of any of the contents of this book.

Trademarks: All terms mentioned in this book that are known to be or are suspected of being trademarks or service marks have been appropriately capitalized. Alpha Books and Penguin Group (USA) Inc. cannot attest to the accuracy of this information. Use of a term in this book should not be regarded as affecting the validity of any trademark or service mark.

Publisher: *Mike Sanders*
Executive Managing Editor: *Billy Fields*
Executive Acquisitions Editor: *Lori Cates Hand*
Development Editors: *Mark Reddin and Christy Wagner*

Senior Production Editor: *Janette Lynn*
Cover/Book Designer: *William Thomas*
Indexer: *Heather McNeill*
Layout: *Ayanna Lacey*
Proofreader: *Laura Caddell*

Contents

Foreword

Aging is an inevitable process that involves an accumulation of changes to the human body over the course of one's lifetime. It's something many of us try to avoid, often through the use of cosmetics or surgery, but to no avail. Some people age gracefully and never appear to grow a day older, and some are not so lucky. But why is this? Is it that some have the gift of great genetics passed down from their parents? Or is it something else? Hippocrates (460–377 B.C.) once said "Let food be thy medicine and medicine be thy food." While this statement was made thousands of years ago, it couldn't be closer to the truth, particularly with regard to aging.

I started my work in the field of aging more than two decades ago as a fellow of the American Institute on Aging. Since that time, I have conducted numerous studies looking at the health benefits of dietary factors on human health. I was amongst the first to show that estrogen and estrogen-like compounds from plants can enhance intestinal calcium absorption; that soy protein may alleviate the symptoms of osteoarthritis; that regular consumption of flaxseed not only lowers cholesterol but more importantly, prevents the formation of fatty lesions, the culprit of arterial plaques; that consumption of a couple apples per day can lower bad cholesterol by 23 percent in a few months; and that the incorporation of a few prunes into our daily diet not only can prevent bone loss but more amazingly can bring back the bone we have already lost.

Fortunately, in recent years, the American Medical Association has stocked all its journals, including its flagship, *JAMA* (*Journal of the American Medical Association*), with articles on such alternative remedies. And though several techniques have withered under scientific scrutiny, others have emerged looking better than mainstream treatments. Hence, isn't it time to change our usual view of medicine as the cultural equivalent of George Washington, while the typical opinion of nutritional intervention is equated with that of Rodney Dangerfield? It is not naive to offer a simple solution to a complex condition. These simple remedies are not really that simple when practiced for an extended period of time. Next time, instead of having an ice cream, try to have a few wedges of watermelon; eat a couple apples or a few ounces of prunes instead of popcorn with added fat; try not to find the closest parking spot when you go to work or shopping; and try to take the stairs instead of the elevator when feasible. Do these things from this day onward, and see the results for yourself.

In *Cheat the Clock,* Margaret Pressler provides an easy-to-understand, yet insightful and scientific, look into how making modest dietary and lifestyle changes can help you look and feel younger, even as you age. This book will be a unique and delightful read for both the lay person and the scientist. Not only does she thoroughly explain the science behind the claims, but she also provides practical tools and suggestions. In her enthusiastic book, Margaret clearly demonstrates the impact we can have on our own health and the rate at which we age through diet, exercise, and other lifestyle factors. This book will provide its readers with a broader understanding of the science behind the aging process and will likely inspire people from all over the world to take control of their health and the way they age.

Bahram H. Arjmandi, PhD, RD

Chair of the Department of Nutrition, Food, and Exercise Sciences, and director of the Center for Advancing Exercise and Nutrition Research on Aging, Florida State University

Preface

We've all met people who look really young for their age. Occasionally, you'll meet someone who looks extraordinary for their age—so much so that you might wonder if they have had any work done or if that hair color is really natural.

I am married to one of those people.

After many years of watching my husband barely age, I decided to try and find out *why* Jim looks so young. I wanted to know if his remarkable youthfulness could tell the rest of us something useful about how to age better ourselves. After all, even though people come in every shape and size and from every conceivable background, we all want to age well.

As a reporter for *The Washington Post*, I was able to take my question to some of the top experts in the field of aging, and the result was a careful look at the science behind my husband's youthful looks. That reporting began a fascinating process of discovery—of groundbreaking lab studies, painstaking academic analyses, and lengthy government reports on the things that make the biggest difference in determining how people age.

That so much research is being done on the subject of aging should be no surprise. The human desire to stay young has been the subject of poetic longing for as long as human thoughts have been recorded. The ancient Greek poet Homer called aging "loathsome." William Shakespeare, 2,400 years later, called it "hideous winter."

Today, thanks to incredible technological and scientific advances, we have high-tech creams to restore our collagen, shoes to firm our fannies, pills to help us lose weight, lasers to even our skin tone, implants to fix our teeth, and, when all else fails, we have liposuction and plastic surgery. As a last resort, we have Photoshop!

From my 2011 *Post* article, I learned that what people really need in order to age well isn't cosmetic or surgical, it's scientific. The discoveries that have been made about aging can do far more than help minimize those fine lines around your eyes. They can help you change your life. Quite simply, you can put into practice the knowledge scientists have amassed to live longer and head into each successive decade with greater health and better looks.

During my research, I was surprised to learn that aging well is not primarily about genetics. Especially as you get older, how you age is far more about what you *do*—your diet, activity level, hobbies, lifestyle, and even your outlook on life. In seeking an answer about Jim, time and again I found that his routine is aligned perfectly with what modern science knows to be the most effective ways to retard the effects of aging. And the impact has been dramatic.

But even more surprising is how easy it has been, for both of us, since I have adopted many of his habits just by living with him. Why aren't more people doing these things? The science on aging is out there. The problem, I realized, is that most people don't know about it—or they don't know how to make it work for *them*.

The scientific community is highly fragmented, with one researcher studying obesity in one lab; another studying skin cells in another; and another tediously testing the impact of sleep cycles, vitamins, or diet on rats in another. Far too often, the eye-opening results of their studies are published, piecemeal, in academic journals such as *Cell* and *Nature,* where few people will see them. Even if they did, they wouldn't understand the medical and scientific jargon used to explain the studies that appear on their pages.

When a few studies on aging do make it into the news cycle, it might be with a small mention in the newspaper. Or if a study comes with really cute pictures of fluffy mice made preternaturally young, it might garner a 2-minute spot on the evening news. Cue the cute tape.

But it's difficult to find one place where all the relevant science is wrapped up together in a simple way that explains what it means to you, and what you can do to remain healthier, more vigorous, and more youthful as you age. That's what this book does.

By learning about the science of aging, you find out the best things you can do to slow down the effects of growing older, whether you're male or female, 30 or 60. Jim's experience is useful not only because it shows the real-life impact such factors can have, but also because he has been able to do it as part of normal life. My husband is not a health and fitness fanatic. He is not a nutrition nut. Yet over the years, he has created an all-natural routine that hews exactly to what you would do if you followed many of the scientific recommendations for keeping the effects of aging at bay.

Most of the scientifically based tips included in this book can noticeably improve your health and well-being, yet they are simple, manageable suggestions. My husband's experience is the jumping-off point, but the science is the path. You don't need to follow a new program to change your entire life, adopt a whole new diet, start a grueling fitness regime, or take a ton of supplements. You just need to know the *best* things to do, and why, and then slowly incorporate them into your existing habits. Start with something as simple as making a slight change to your bedtime routine, for example, or trying a new kind of snack. Some suggestions might be a bigger change for you, but overall, they're probably a lot less burdensome than you might expect—and far more effective.

The secret to success lies in your time frame. Because aging itself takes time, even if you move toward better age-retarding habits in tiny steps, the changes add up over months and years to make a big difference. How can that be? Because what you do as you get older affects how you age more than what you did when you were young—even more, in some cases, than your genetics. If the impact of what you do is magnified as you age, then a small behavior that might make no difference to a 20-something makes a bigger difference to a 35-year-old and a much bigger difference to someone who is 55.

The importance of this can't be overstated; it means that once you're in your 40s or 50s, rather than being too late to affect the way you age, you've actually reached the point when you can influence it the most. So whatever your age right now, it's more important than ever that you know what to do and then make a few easy changes to your life so you can start reaping the rewards for years to come.

The information in this book comes in three forms: what the science says about why it works, suggestions for ways to incorporate the change into your routine, and in many cases the real-life experience of my husband and how he's done it. What makes this structure valuable is that if you know something has scientifically proven benefits, you're more likely to stick with it. If you stick with it, you'll begin to notice that it's making a difference. And once you've noticed the improvement, you'll want to do another small thing and then another. Keep this book handy! With any luck, you'll eventually find yourself in a new place, physically and psychologically, feeling better and younger than you've felt in years and amazed that the transition was so painless. This is the transformation I have watched Jim experience.

It's important to note that the focus of this book is long term. It's not going to help you lose 20 pounds before your reunion. It's not a diet. My hope is that as you read the book, and gain a true understanding of the science of aging, you will feel empowered to make targeted changes to your own life. The suggestions in these pages are designed to be easy to incorporate into your daily life for good, not just for a few weeks or months. It's about finding new approaches you can embrace so they become part of the way you live.

Making changes this way is not nearly as hard as going on a diet or starting a new fitness program, but nonetheless, they still may not be an easy sell. America has a love affair with the quick fix, whether it's a carb-free diet that squeezes 10 pounds off your frame in 2 weeks, a pill that lowers your blood pressure, or a machine that promises the effect of a full workout in just 5 minutes. Look at the way we celebrate the contestants on *The Biggest Loser* reality show—the winner each week is the person who loses the most weight.

But plans like that are almost always impossible to keep up. Like everyone else, I've joined gyms and stopped going; gone on diets and given up. The fact is, most people simply can't change all their habits in one fell swoop and stick with it—at least, not without the help of Hollywood handlers or a hefty paycheck. America's steadily expanding waistlines and growing health-care problems are proof of that.

But you *do* want to age well, so why not try a different approach? Don't think about all the issues you may want to fix right now, whether it's losing weight or exercising more or eating better, healthier food. Instead, think about how you want to feel 10 or 15 years from now and work toward *that* goal. If you start making just small changes now, and let them grow over time, when 10 years have passed, you'll have made a big difference in the way you feel. But if you keep doing nothing to improve your long-term health, you are guaranteed to look and feel 10 or 15 years older than you do now. Those years are going to pass anyway, so if you can do just a few things scientifically proven to help you feel younger even as you get older, you'll have found a way to cheat the clock.

Maybe it's hard to think that far in advance, so start with an exercise that's a little closer to home. Close your eyes and picture where you'll be in 5 years. Maybe your kids will be in high school. Maybe you'll be nearing retirement age. Maybe your mortgage will be paid off. Maybe that kitchen renovation will finally be finished!

Now, picture yourself at that same place in time, still 5 years older, but *feeling* younger and healthier. Which one do you want? The answer is easy. So is the path to get there. My husband Jim is the proof.

Acknowledgments

I could not have written this book without the help of many people, especially, of course, my husband, Jim, who gamely went along with this project from the beginning. Besides letting me probe and expose every facet of his care and feeding routines, he was instrumental in helping shape the concept of the book—and make more than a few word choices as my partner and sounding board. Throughout the reporting and writing of the book, I also got terrific, fast research help from Judy Park, whose responsiveness helped me keep up with a very quick turnaround schedule. My agent and friend Richard Levy, more than anyone, is responsible for making my vision for the book a reality, and I can't thank him enough for believing in me, trusting me, and putting himself on the line for me. I must also express my deep gratitude to the editors at *The Washington Post* for supporting my pursuit of this project, especially Tracy Grant, Peter Perl, and Shirley Carswell; what a fantastic place to work for the past 23 years. I am equally indebted to the numerous brilliant scientists who dropped what they were doing to explain their research to me; their insights and efforts were—and are—invaluable. Of course, creating a finished product also required tremendous support and effort from the great staff at Alpha Books, especially Mike Sanders, Lori Cates Hand, and my editors Mark Reddin and Christy Wagner. Thanks also to Michael Katigbak of the Mandarin Oriental Hotel for letting us use a beautiful suite to shoot our portrait. On a personal note, I want to thank my three children for being so understanding when, for several months, I couldn't be there as much as I wished. And thank you to my mother, who did whatever she could for me, even when it was a terrible time for her (and who was also a great editor), and to my late father, for being so excited about my first book, which he sadly never got to read.

Part 1

The New Science on Aging

An Introduction to Jim

Nearly 10 years ago, with two little kids in tow, my husband and I wandered lazily through the midway at the West Virginia State Fair. The smell of smoking nuts, popcorn, and cotton candy wafted through the air, with blinking lights and ringing bells completing the sensory overload. Among the food counters, rickety rides, and can't-win game stalls was a weathered, red-faced man just outside a small wooden booth.

"Guess your age within 2 years!" the sign read. "$2"

How could we lose? We sidled up to the booth behind a pair of friendly looking, middle-aged women who were laughing nervously as they waited for the guessing game to begin. The carnie was eyeing one of the women carefully. Then he wrote something on a tiny yellow sticky note in his hand and gave it to her. She groaned loudly, the way you do when you've just lost $2 to a carnie at a fair.

"How old are you?" the carnie asked. "51!" she said, incredulous. And she and her friend walked away. He had nailed it. Undeterred, we moved up to the booth, and I pushed Jim forward, ahead of me and the stroller. "Can you guess his age?" I asked. The carnie looked my husband over, squinting in the sun, examining his hair, face, and body. Then he glanced over at me and the young 'uns, scratched his pencil on another sticky note, and handed it over. I craned to see what he wrote.

"37," it read. We won! "I'm 55," my husband said, smiling. The carnie recoiled a bit, clearly caught off guard. "Well, now," he said, "I think I'm gonna have to see your license for that one."

My husband pulled out his wallet and handed over his license, which the carnie inspected for a while before handing it back with another long, hard look at Jim.

"*Damn,*" he said. "You look *good.*"

Asking the Question

That my husband looks good for his age has long been the subject of shocked, humorous, and disbelieving comments, although the one from the West Virginia carnival still ranks among our favorites.

But as Jim has moved into his 60s, those comments have intensified because somehow he has managed to age even *less* in the past decade than in the one before. Now, although I'm 17 years his junior and firmly in my 40s, few people ever think there's any age difference between us at all. And when Jim runs into old classmates or co-workers he hasn't seen in years, his unchanging appearance is almost always the first thing they talk about.

"How do you do it?" is the constant question.

I had always assumed Jim's remarkable lack of aging was the result of singularly good genes, with perhaps a little boost from that vibrant young wife of his. Because he's just an ordinary guy and not some health and fitness guru, I had never really thought about it beyond that.

But as more and more people asked, he began to regularly explain the particular things he does to take care of himself—what he eats, the way he exercises, his lifestyle, his personal-care habits, and nutrition. Listening to him talk about this over and over, it dawned on me that over the years he has developed a pretty great routine. He's done it slowly and, frankly, quite effortlessly, so I never paid much attention to it. But the more he talked about it, the more I wondered if he was actually having more of an impact on his looks and vitality than I'd thought.

As a reporter for *The Washington Post,* I took my question to some of the top experts in the fields of aging. I told them about Jim, sent pictures, and provided a complete rundown of his habits—good and bad. I was honest about it. The chocolate-chip cookies he adores, and eats daily after dinner, went into the "bad" category, for example. Then I posed the $10,000 question: is it genetics, or is it something he does?

I've always been interested in health and nutrition, but what unfolded as I reported this story, and beyond, was far more than I expected. An incredible amount of research is going on about aging and the factors that affect it. As I learned about these studies and research, I found that Jim happens to do an amazing number of things known to stop the effects of aging. It's not just that he's exercising, it's that he's exercising the right way. It's not just that he's at a good weight, it's how he got there. In ways big and small, he is right on the money.

Doing so many things right—exactly right—at the right time in his life, I learned, was the main reason behind Jim's phenomenal youthfulness. Scientifically speaking, the correlation between these factors and aging well is so strong that scientists could say, with certainty, that Jim has had a huge impact on the way he looks and feels for his age.

I wrote a piece on what I had learned for *The Washington Post*'s Health section, and it quickly became the most-read story on the paper's website, drawing huge traffic. My email inbox filled with questions and comments. Never mind that many of those emails included the accusation that—for sure!—Jim had either dyed his hair or had plastic surgery. Neither is true; he is 100 percent natural, I explained to the skeptics. Some accepted my response, while others just wouldn't believe it, even as they offered compliments to him for looking, and feeling, so good for his age.

You're probably thinking Jim is blessed with good genes; to be honest, that's what everyone says when they see him. And to some degree, they—and you—are probably right. It's likely that Jim's genes have predisposed him to age well, although what that lucky cocktail of genetic markers might be—indeed, whether he even has them—is something scientists can't identify, at least not yet. What scientists *do* know, for sure, is that if he didn't take care of himself the way he does, he simply would not look nearly as youthful as he does, nor be as healthy, genes or no genes. As one top aging exert told me, when it comes to aging, genes are largely what you make of them.

"You don't get the gene of being younger, you get the gene that allows you, if you do the right things, to slow down your aging process," said Luigi Ferrucci, scientific director at the National Institute on Aging, part of the National Institutes of Health. "What we call it is gene-environmental interaction."

In other words, you've got the genes you've got, but you can influence them, and more than you think. Even more important, the changes you make can be passed on to your offspring. This compelling field of emerging science is called epigenetics. The more you know about it, the more it makes you think about how you're treating your body.

But what really pushed me to write this book is that my husband was able to bring about this huge change in his life—and by extension, my life and the lives of our three children—so easily.

How Jim Got Here

Jim is a regular guy. Sometimes he goes a week or two without finding time to exercise, especially if he's caught a cold brought home from school. He wouldn't, and couldn't, run a marathon, in part because he pretty much dislikes running. And he has a very busy, stressful law practice that keeps him at the office 6 days a week. Add three kids to the mix, and you get the idea. He may be a little older than most parents with elementary-school-age children, but in every other way, he's a typical dad without a lot of extra time for himself.

I don't mean to minimize his efforts when it comes to aging well, of course. He is purposeful about taking care of himself. But where fitness and health used to feel like work, they're now just a part of the way he lives. And if Jim can do it, anyone can.

So before we look at the science of aging in subsequent chapters, let's look at exactly how, and why, Jim developed his age-defying routine.

In the winter of 1969, Jim was in his senior year in college at Villanova University outside Philadelphia. He rushed back from a long weekend away to get to a class that was from 10 to noon on Tuesday only to find the teacher was absent. As everyone was milling around, figuring out what to do with a spare 2 hours, one student was asking everyone what lottery number they had gotten and checking it in the newspaper.

It was the first year a lottery system had been used for the draft for the Vietnam War. Your lottery number was tied, randomly, to your birth date, with numbers from 1 to 366. Those with lower numbers would be drafted first. Those with numbers in the middle faced uncertainty about being drafted. And those with the highest numbers would probably not be drafted.

"What's your lottery number?" The student asked Jim as he was heading out of the classroom.

"I don't know," Jim replied. The numbers had been released the night before, and he hadn't seen a paper to check. (Imagine how fast that kind of news would spread today!)

"What's your birthday?" Jim's classmate persisted.

"August 8," Jim said. The kid looked down at the newspaper.

"Oh," he said. "You got 48."

It was a shock. Jim had been accepted to law school, but with such a low lottery number, he was certain to be drafted.

In the fall, right on cue, he was called to report for a military physical. He was anxious that day, of course, as he was ushered through the health assessment process at the coliseum in downtown Philadelphia. After several hours, he was told to sit at one desk in a long row of desks while a stern-looking doctor evaluated his results, which showed that Jim's blood pressure was high. The doctor told him he needed to get further testing over 3 days, which he did through a private doctor. This resulted in a 6-month deferment.

When Jim went back to the coliseum 6 months later, he was ushered along the same long row of desks and happened to get the same unfriendly doctor. He looked over Jim's records again, and took his blood pressure. Then he looked at Jim and said, "Son, have you ever seen a doctor for this problem? I'm recommending you for a permanent deferment."

And that was it. Jim would not go to Vietnam; he would go to law school.

"I never found out what my blood pressure was that day," Jim says now. "They didn't tell me. Actually, I'm kind of glad I don't know."

You might think Jim would have taken this news as a reason to actually go to a doctor to treat his blood pressure. But he didn't. "When you're young, you don't think about things like that," he said. "I really thought it was because I was nervous being there."

It wasn't until 2 years later that Jim got a real wakeup call. The summer after his second year in law school in Boston, he applied for a job to operate a forklift truck on a construction site. He needed a physical to get the job, and once again, his blood pressure was high, and this time, he couldn't chalk it up to nerves. The doctor gave him a prescription to treat it, but after a month, Jim stopped taking the medication. "I didn't want to be on drugs," he said. He wanted to find a natural way to bring down his blood pressure.

Jim started researching natural ways to control hypertension, and based on the information he found, he decided to stop eating red meat. While living in Boston, he would go to the Faneuil Hall market and buy fresh fish, inexpensively. He also ate chicken and a lot of beans. "I ate really well," he said. "I remember I didn't have any money to spend on food. But I figured out how to make things that were good."

By the time Jim was out of law school and had moved to Washington, D.C., as a new lawyer, his blood pressure was down to the normal range. He did not continue to shun red meat completely, but the experience earlier in his life changed his attitude about it. "It just made me feel, instinctively, that it wasn't doing my body any good," he said. "So I only ate it occasionally. And when I did eat it, I tried to only eat red meat that was really lean."

From Then to Now

He didn't know it at the time, but cutting back on red meat was the first step to protecting his health and youthfulness for years to come. Since then, many studies have come out explaining the detrimental effect of consuming red meat on health and aging, although not everything about this interaction is fully understood. All together, though, the evidence clearly points to a strong connection not only between health and red meat consumption, but between aging and red meat. (I talk more about this connection, and ways to tailor your diet around it, later in the book.)

This early experience set Jim on a course of *mindfulness* about what he eats, which is essential for anyone who wants to navigate a world full of unhealthy messages and choices. Mindfulness does not mean denial or counting calories—it's really about listening to the signals from your body, good and bad, and following them. This kind of awareness was forced on Jim because of a medical condition, and because he chose to treat his nascent blood pressure condition naturally, if possible. That forced him to pay closer attention to how he actually felt.

It sounds simple, but awareness *is* really the easiest and perhaps smallest step available to start living in a way that values your long-term health and welfare and takes it where you want to go. Anyone can learn to think this way. People often ignore signals from their own bodies because they assume they're a natural part of growing old, or are something that will pass. Or often they believe the remedy would be so unpleasant (lots of exercise! no dessert!) that they opt to ignore it. So in this book, I talk a lot about what signals your body is sending—maybe exhaustion or heartburn, for example—and what they mean, as well as the often tiny adjustments you can make to help push away those signals and put your body on a path to long-term health and vitality.

A lot of this may just sound like starting good habits and stopping bad ones—and wouldn't we all do that if we could? Well, yes, but the fact is, bad habits *can* be broken and good habits *can* be encouraged if you approach it right, as Jim has. Being aware of your motivations and the psychology of habit formation is a big part of the battle, and this book helps you identify—and diminish—the role of your typical triggers and excuses so you can start tackling habits you'd most like to ditch or develop. For my husband, establishing good habits was easier than quitting bad ones, but he has been largely successful at both (except maybe the chocolate-chip cookies), primarily because he has approached it with a long-term goal. When he gets off track, it's not a game changer—he doesn't give up. Getting back on track is what matters.

When it comes to helping your body handle year after year of age-inducing stress, work, anxiety, and heartache, it's far better to have a few good habits you keep coming back to than to take on too much and throw in the towel the first time you fail.

For Jim, having this kind of awareness was the fundamental step that allowed him to slowly build a routine of model antiaging habits. He didn't start out to with the goal of having no health problems and almost no wrinkles at the age of 64; he did these things because he followed his body's signals, which grew louder with each subsequent tweaking of his routine. But he came to appreciate—as I have now—the long-term benefits.

A good analogy is remodeling your house: once you paint the walls, you realize how shabby the floors look. Those floors may bug you, but you live with them. Eventually, though, you just don't want to live with those floors anymore, so as soon as you have the money, replacing them becomes a priority.

Over the years, Jim has remodeled his walls and replaced his floors primarily because it felt better to live that way. And as we all know, taking care of your house makes it last longer and helps retain its value.

A Road Map to Aging Well

In the upcoming chapters, you learn about what Jim has done that has made such an impact on his health and looks, and how the latest science can help you live better and longer, too. But in a nutshell, the following sections outline the primary areas in which Jim has achieved an optimal level of antiaging benefits over many years.

Nutrition

Jim's diet already leaned heavily toward lean meats and fish, but he has been gradually eating less of the bad things (like sweets and chips, for example) and more good things. Dark green vegetables, fruit, nuts, and—this is a biggie—whole grains are now staples in his diet. Scientists are learning more all the time about the significant role such nutrient- and antioxidant-rich foods play in slowing the aging process.

Jim also has been taking moderate vitamin E supplements since he was in law school, around the same time he began treating his high blood pressure. Vitamin E is a powerful antioxidant vital to the human body, yet many Americans don't get nearly the amount they need. In these pages, I share the latest science on this subject—some of which is controversial—and what it means for you. Even if you don't take vitamin E supplements—and the latest studies suggest higher-dose supplements could be harmful—I show you natural ways to boost the amount of vitamin E in your diet.

It's hard to discuss nutrition without talking about weight, of course, and although a tremendous amount is still not known about aging and nutrition, scientists do know there's a direct link between obesity and premature aging. Jim has never been an especially thin guy, but he's never been overweight, either. The first important step in achieving this over many years was not ignoring his weight and its slight fluctuations from week to week or month to month. He has developed an array of useful tricks to get himself to eat a little less whenever necessary—after the holidays or a vacation, for example—which he employed to lose 10 pounds over 2 years without dieting.

If you need to lose weight, the best way to do so when it comes to aging is to lose it slowly. Americans don't much like the idea of losing weight over a long period of time, but if your goal is aging well, the tortoise had it right: slow and steady wins the race.

Exercise

Talk about an on-again off-again love affair. Jim was once captain of his hockey team and rowed on the crew team—a true college athlete. In the two decades after college, he stayed fit with tennis and sometimes went running.

But like most people, "I remember periods in which I exercised, and periods in which I didn't," he said. There was a long stretch in his late 40s and early 50s when he didn't exercise much at all, thanks to an incredibly busy and growing law practice. But that changed when he noticed that just a little bit of exercise, even 20 minutes a couple times a week, helped him handle the physical as well as emotional demands of having young children. He couldn't help the fact that he had his first baby at age 50, and he wanted to meet the demands of the task. Coming home and vegging out with a glass of wine and a pile of cheese puffs wasn't working for him anymore.

So the very moderate exercise Jim began diligently doing 10 years ago wasn't so much about looking better or meeting some fitness ideal. It was really about feeling less tired and more focused so he could enjoy his young family even after a long day at work. That now-ingrained habit was fairly easy to accomplish, and it has been essential to his health today.

According to scientific studies, moderate exercise is the absolute best way to thwart the effects of aging. And the reverse is true: getting no exercise is the single worst thing you can do if you want to age well. But getting a lot of exercise conveys comparatively fewer benefits than lighter workouts. So the sweet spot is moderate exercise— something you can accomplish if you let yourself start slowly and build up to it, and this book lays out various manageable options.

Exercise does not have to be an all-or-nothing concept. Even if you take a few brisk walks a week, and throw in some sit-ups, push-ups, or other weight-bearing exercises, it will pay a huge dividend in a few years, and probably much sooner.

Personal Care

This stuff really matters, but you don't need expensive lotions and facials. All you need are a few good habits and a commitment to the basics.

Jim has been using the same drugstore brand of moisturizer, Olay, since he was in his 20s. He flosses every single night without fail—an underemphasized habit that can have a big impact on your overall health. He doesn't get too much sun, but he does get enough sleep. He goes to the doctor when something's wrong, and he gets a physical every year.

These are such simple steps, yet compelling scientific evidence shows that these minimal efforts pay a huge dividend in health and looks for years to come. If you have even basic health insurance, none of these things will cost you much in time or money. But each one is an important investment in your future well-being, and they really don't take a lot of effort.

It may take an attitude adjustment, but knowing why you're doing these things—understanding the science behind them—should help with that.

Lifestyle

If you have a hobby, nurture it. Better yet, if you have a spouse, boyfriend, child, parent, or friend who has the same hobby, do it together. Studies show that finding something you enjoy doing and sharing it with someone has a big effect on your aging process. It doesn't have to be intense, though.

Jim, for example, enjoys architecture, and we often walk around old neighborhoods and admire houses, trying to squirrel away ideas for our own house. He also likes shopping and has a wife and two daughters who are only too happy to come along! But his biggest hobby is photography, and although he does this largely alone, he gets enormous joy from displaying his photographs and giving them as gifts. Studies show that staying intellectually engaged and socially connected has a powerful impact on preserving vitality and youthfulness.

Even as I write about the wide range of things Jim has done through the years that, according to aging experts, have contributed to his incredible youthfulness, I am amazed at the length of the list. Because I live with him, and I know—thankfully—he's not obsessive or weird about any of it, I find it almost hard to believe he has so effortlessly pulled together so many good habits and choices. It has unfolded so slowly and naturally as to be virtually unnoticeable in our lives, except, of course, it's far from inconsequential because everyone in our family has benefitted from his tremendous vitality even at age 64. And let's face it, those good habits are rubbing off on the rest of us.

As I've poked and prodded into his habits and then promptly turned around and shared them with total strangers (aging experts, but still), Jim has been a trooper. It's one thing for me to ask the question about why my husband looks so young; it's another for him to go along with it. I started out wanting to know what his habits were doing for him from a scientific perspective. He was motivated by the desire to let other people know that, frankly, it's not that hard and they can do it, too.

A big part of Jim's success has come from being smart about aging and encouraging himself to get smarter—to find out what works and what he should do. That knowledge has helped him make better choices in many areas of his life, with fantastic results. Now it's your turn.

To Age or
Not to Age?

What do you think about when you picture yourself getting older? Do you think of gaining wisdom and security and finally having the time to do the things you've always wanted? Or do you think of illness, infirmity, and loneliness? Are you rocking in a chair or rocking a new you?

Your answers are surprisingly important. Studies have shown that the way you view aging when you're still young plays an important role in determining how well you're going to fare as the years actually pass by.

Knowing that, you might be a little concerned about your answers to those questions about aging. If you'd like to change your answers, you can. First, though, you need to learn a little more about how and why aging actually happens. By understanding the aging process, you'll be less afraid to face it and more empowered to control the way it happens to you.

What follows in this chapter is an explanation of the latest scientific knowledge of the aging process. I've tried to present this fairly technical information as simply as possible, without a lot of distracting scientific terminology. Learning about this research is important because if you want to make a difference to the way you age, you need to know what's going on inside you, not just in terms of digestion or metabolism, but in terms of cellular function.

The concepts outlined in this chapter may be complex, but they underlie all the useful scientific research aimed at helping you do the right things that will allow you to age better, which is the focus of the rest of the book. To really get the most out of all this, you need to start with the tough stuff. And if nothing else, all this scientific information will leave you with an incredible respect for the almost unimaginable complexity of human life!

Aging by Design

Aging brings a cascade of changes to the body and mind that are familiar to everyone, even if you haven't experienced them yet (or haven't admitted to it, anyway!). Children inherently know their parents are older than they are and their grandparents are older still, and usually very early on they learn that somewhere up there at grandparent age or beyond, people die. This rather unpleasant ending to the aging process makes it a subject many people don't like to think about or discuss. It's just something we have to live with and navigate around the best we can. It's unavoidable, yet we all want to avoid it.

But scientists take a less emotional view: aging is a result of evolution and the natural selection process. As a species, we have evolved to be at our healthiest when we're young and in our reproductive years. From the perspective of evolution, there was no benefit to keeping us around into old age. If anything, there was every reason *not* to have us around, being another mouth to feed.

So evolution allowed us to start falling apart around middle age—if you could escape the sabertooth tiger that long. It's only been in very recent years, from a human-history perspective, that we've been able to outsmart the pressures of natural selection and reach our 70s and beyond. It will take even more effort to add another decade or two to that typical lifespan.

Now that a huge portion of the population is heading into middle age and beyond, there's growing interest in the science of aging. Although scientists are quick to say there's still a great deal they don't understand about aging, and the funding for aging research is paltry— less than 1 percent of the entire budget of the National Institutes of Health—it is nevertheless true that the knowledge base is evolving at a dramatic pace. And much of what's being discovered has the power to transform the way everyone thinks about growing older and, therefore, the way they live now.

Here's the single most important message from all this research: it's becoming abundantly clear that you have a great deal of control over your future years. So if you didn't have such a favorable answer to the question at the start of this chapter, you can take heart. Aging is not immutable, as you may think, even if your parents didn't do it so well!

This was a surprise to me; before I began delving into the latest science on aging, I was pretty certain my husband's good fortune was the result of good genes. I was surprised to find out that's not the case—at least not primarily.

"There is a lot of research that shows that about 25 percent of the age you're going to live to is determined by your genes. That means the other 75 percent is not," says biologist Dr. Steven Austad, interim director of the Barshop Institute for Longevity and Aging Studies at the University of Texas Health Science Center San Antonio. "That means there is a lot of room to affect how you age."

In other words, if you want to age well, you have to make it happen, because your genes aren't going to do it for you. But the good news is you *can* make it happen. Now that scientists know so much about aging, excellent information is available to help you do it better.

> "There is a lot of research that shows that about 25 percent of the age you're going to live to is determined by your genes. That means the other 75 percent is not."

The Mystery of Aging

Researchers like Dr. Austad are toiling away in laboratories trying to untangle the big questions about aging: what, exactly, causes us to age, why do some people age better than others, and what can regular people do to stay healthy and youthful through the years? What motivates these experts is this simple fact: aging is the single biggest risk factor for 70 percent of the diseases that affect Americans. By improving, or slowing down, the aging process, we can minimize the impact of many of the world's most feared medical conditions. It's not just cosmetic; there are really good reasons to try to keep the clock from ticking so fast.

But what is the "aging process"? Is it wrinkled skin, a weakening skeleton, and a slowing mind? No, it's far more complex than that. Much of the aging process, in fact, is invisible; the part we see and associate with aging is just one piece of it. Figuring out what makes us age requires scientists with advanced degrees in such fields as biochemistry, neurology, psychology, oncology, and pharmacology who can look for clues and cures at the cellular level.

Dr. Austad, for example, is trying to figure out how to make life better for longer by delving into the mysteries of enzymes and proteins with unpronounceable names, genetic signaling systems, and the superior aging skills of some nonhuman species. He is convinced we have not reached the upper limit of human lifespan, which right now stands at 122, or the highest age any person on Earth is known to have reached.

To most people, aging is just something you do, like sleeping at night or waking in the morning. You may wonder, for example, what causes wrinkles—or more likely, what makes them disappear!—but scientists are asking much bigger questions: Do we have to age? Is there a mechanism that controls the decline? They are trying to answer these questions by looking at what makes our very cells wear out and die within our bodies, even as we remain living. They want to know why we become susceptible to so many age-related diseases later in life, such as diabetes, heart disease, and cancer.

One way to answer those questions is to look at species that don't age the way we do. Some of the research conducted today seems like it could hardly be relevant to humans: scientists study clownfish, yeast, and microscopic worms, for example. Dr. Austad also likes to study bats and is currently working with clams—specifically, a species of clam that can live for more than 500 years.

"Most people don't know this, but clams have a beating heart," Dr. Austad says. "So here you can hold in your hand a heart that has been beating since before Shakespeare was born, and that's kind of a mind-blowing phenomenon. We're really interested in figuring out how they do it."

Until just a few decades ago, research on aging was largely descriptive, identifying what happens during the aging process by observing and documenting the cellular changes that come with advancing age. This has been done in exquisite detail in small animals, such as lab mice, and even in the simplest organisms, such as yeast and microscopic worms called *C. elegans*. These worms aren't much to look at, but they are much appreciated in aging labs for their 2-week lifespan, which gives researchers nearly instant results when they make genetic or environmental changes that affect the organism.

Today, aging research is moving into the more time-consuming and complex study of aging in mammals, primates, and humans. Scientists are investigating the interplay of genes, proteins, enzymes, and micronutrients, as well as outside environmental factors, including diet and lifestyle, that all seem to affect aging in different ways.

The discoveries are growing exponentially, each one getting tantalizingly closer to the answer.

Aging Answers

"I am sure that there is one underlying mechanism of aging," says Dr. Luigi Ferrucci, scientific director of the National Institute on Aging at the National Institutes of Health outside Washington, D.C. "There is a director of the orchestra that is tuning all the sounds together, and then at some point ... that harmony gets lost."

Dr. Ferrucci's career is dedicated to solving the mysteries of this symphony, most recently running a large population study of people from the Baltimore area, called the Baltimore Longitudinal Study of Aging (BLSA), which began in 1958 with rolling admission. Individuals admitted to the group must have exceptional health upon entering and must agree to be followed with surveys and examinations, even genetically, throughout their lives. Many of the original participants have since died, so currently 1,300 people are enrolled in the study.

The high scientific standards of the BLSA have made it a gold mine of significant data scientists can use to study normal aging and what affects it, as well as age-related diseases and what precipitates them.

Healthspan, Not Lifespan

Through all these discoveries about aging, the focus of aging researchers has shifted. Where scientists once talked about extending our lifespan, now they use a different word to encapsulate their goals: *healthspan*. No one wants to live to be 90 if they're going to be sick, dependent, and incoherent for their last 10 years or more. So when people talk about "living longer" or having a "longer lifespan," they really mean having more years of relatively good health. This important difference shifts the focus from increasing longevity to preventing age-related diseases. And the latter largely depends on how you live when you're younger.

I took my husband with me when I met with Dr. Ferrucci at his offices, on the seventh floor of a nondescript office building at the headquarters of the National Institutes of Health, a massive development where 19,000 people go to work every day. I had given Dr. Ferrucci the background about Jim when I wrote my *Post* story, but when we finally reached his office months later, I was surprised that he registered no reaction at all upon seeing Jim in person.

Even Dr. Austad, after seeing a picture of Jim, had this to say in an email: "Goodness. You might give up the newspaper business and make a living on the carnie circuit taking money from the 'bet I can guess your age' booths." (I didn't tell him we've already done that!)

I realized later that Dr. Ferrucci's reaction to Jim was merely scientific. He studies aging in people, and he knows the behaviors that make a difference, especially in the areas of nutrition. So to him, Jim was just another example of what works, as he has seen many times before throughout his career. What he really cares about, and what he's trying to figure out, is *why*.

Population studies like the BLSA can answer a lot of questions about the impact of what you do, and about the interaction of your genes and the environment. But the real answers have to come from inside cells and understanding how they live, behave, and die. Just as aging affects your physical well-being in many overt ways, aging begins with many less-obvious changes in your cells and their functions—changes that are directly influenced by what you do. Scientists are focusing their efforts on the role these cellular changes play in human aging and how you can stop them.

But scientists aren't the only people who should know this information—you should, too. When you know what's going on inside your body, you know what to do to help it. For example, if you knew (and you probably do) that broccoli was good for you, you might try to eat it now and then. But what if you knew that scientists have discovered a chemical compound in broccoli that attaches to your DNA and helps suppress genes that cause cancer? That would make you reach for the green stuff more often, wouldn't it?

> "What if you knew that scientists have discovered a chemical compound in broccoli that attaches to your DNA and helps suppress genes that cause cancer?"

If you decide, as my husband did, to make changes that will help you live a longer, healthier life, you can do it one of two ways. You can either act it on faith—believing that the outcome will be what you expect 5 or 10 years down the road—or you can make an effort to understand the science of aging and how the choices you make affect you at the cellular level. The latter is far more motivating!

Six Sources of Aging

Scientists have honed in on several key areas of cellular change that seem to have the biggest influence on aging, and many of them, such as Dr. Ferrucci, are convinced that the interplay of these factors affects how and why we age.

Age-related changes are enormously complex, in part because cellular-level reactions occur slightly differently in each one of us as we grow from child to parent to grandparent. Researchers are trying to untangle the clues, of course, but many aging experts believe the best treatment for age-related decline is, and will always be, prevention.

Pills and medical treatments may do some good as you age, but they will never be as effective as taking steps now, when you're younger, to prevent age-related decline in the first place. Alzheimer's disease is a great example. It's been increasingly documented that certain lifestyle factors can prevent or delay the onset of this horrible, progressive disease. But once it's been diagnosed, it's irreversible.

To really take care of yourself now, though, you need to know what to do. You need to know how your body works. You need knowledge. Research psychologists who work on aging and health issues spend a lot of time studying people's motivation to change and reactions to health issues because what people do to affect their health is just as important as whatever conditions they may have or get. These scientists find that people who know what's going on inside them feel empowered to change and improve. But most people don't have a clue how their bodies work, even when it comes to some of the basics.

Increasingly, universities are beginning to offer science-based health courses for members of the community, not just students, as part of their ongoing education programs. Distinguished researchers, eager to get their lab findings out to the public, are writing books and offering classes and even online courses and seminars. They see, in their working groups and labs, how enlightening it is when real people learn how a particular system actually works and what it responds to, or how a single behavior change can help, and why.

Stanford lecturer and author Dr. Kelly McGonigal calls this movement "science help." She teaches continuing education courses at Stanford with names such as The New Science of Surviving and Thriving in the Modern World and is starting online seminars.

"Understanding the science creates motivation, or it creates insight that allows people to change when they're more educated about the workings of their brain and body," she says.

In this chapter, you learn about the six main factors now known by scientists to be major contributors to aging. Much of the rest of the book looks at how different behaviors and lifestyles affect these processes. Once you've got this information, you can make a judgment about what you'd like to improve and have solid, scientifically based information to act upon.

I've tried to present these complex topics as simply as possible because this is essential reading: to get the most of the advice in this book, you need to know these basic facts about how your body ages. Chances are, as you're reading, you'll come across numerous facts that will make you say, "So *that's* why that happens!"

These are the aging processes:

- Cell stress
- Cell death and other changes in the cell's lifecycle
- Shortening of the protective caps on our DNA, called telomeres
- Abnormal proteins
- Genetics
- Epigenetics, or environmentally influenced changes in how some genes are expressed

If you understand these concepts, you've taken a big step toward influencing the way you age.

Stressed-Out Cells

The human body is an efficient machine that needs energy to operate. But the process of making that energy creates pollution inside your cells, just like a car engine burning gasoline. When that engine is running perfectly with the right kind of fuel, the pollution is kept in check; but when your engine gets old or the fuel isn't perfect, the noxious waste produced goes from the equivalent of a tiny puff to full-on smog. That pollution causes all the harmful effects you'd expect from a red-level air-quality alert.

This cellular pollution has a familiar name: *free radicals*. Free radicals have been widely implicated as a main cause of aging, and now marketing messages everywhere are promoting foods that fight free radical damage. But it is not that simple.

The energy your body uses is manufactured by little structures inside your cells called *mitochondria,* which have a number of jobs, including regulating how cells develop and even how they die.

But their main function is to be the power plants for your body, constantly converting the sugars from the food you eat into a form of chemical energy called ATP (adenosine triphosphate), which your cells can then use to keep your heart pumping, your brain thinking, your lungs breathing, and your muscles moving. "All the energy you get is packed in this high-energy molecule that powers everything," explains Dr. Bruce Ames, professor of biochemistry and molecular biology at the University of California, Berkeley.

Like a burning fire, mitochondria must consume oxygen to turn food sugars into ATP. When they're young and healthy, they do this with incredible efficiency that produces very little waste or pollution. But during this process, some oxygen molecules don't get used properly, setting off a destructive chain reaction that, ultimately, leads to aging.

The structure of the oxygen molecule allows free radicals to form. Inside its nucleus are pairs of electrons, one rotating in one direction, creating a microscopic magnetic field, and the other electron rotating in the opposite direction, creating an opposite magnetic field. Those two magnetic fields balance each other, leaving the oxygen molecule stable, with no magnetic force.

During normal metabolism, as your mitochondria are converting your tuna sandwich, say, into ATP, the occasional oxygen molecule loses an electron. That leaves the oxygen molecule off-kilter because a single, unpaired electron is left spinning away on its own, creating a magnetic force in one direction. The molecule dances around frantically, trying to find another electron with an opposite magnetic field to pair up with so it can become stable again.

This molecule slams around inside the cell like a pinball in a machine, damaging almost everything it runs into—the mitochondria, proteins, cell membranes, and even your DNA. It may manage to snag an electron from another molecule, and it will become stable again, but then that other molecule becomes unstable and begins its own crazy, destructive search for another electron to pair with. These unstable molecules missing an electron are the *free radicals*. The chain reaction of damage these free radicals cause, molecule by molecule, is called *oxidative stress*.

> "Some oxygen molecules don't get used properly, setting off a destructive chain reaction that, ultimately, leads to aging."

"When you have free radical damage, all hell breaks loose," says Dr. Maret Traber, professor of nutrition at Oregon State University (OSU) and a researcher at the OSU Linus Pauling Institute, which investigates the role of nutrition and micronutrients in health and aging. "How do you describe a bomb falling on a building? There are charred pieces, broken pieces."

If this kind of oxidative damage went unchecked, none of us would live very long; our cells would become so badly damaged they'd no longer function. But the body has a well-honed defense system to gobble up free radicals and break the chain reaction of damage from this so-called oxidization. These safety systems are enzymes and proteins whose sole function is to act as *anti*oxidants. They lend an electron to the unstable molecule so it will calm down and stop damaging the cell from the inside. These antioxidants, with unmemorable names such as superoxide dismutase and catalase, are critical to keeping your cells from spiraling out of control.

The damage caused by oxidative stress gets cleaned up by another system of repair enzymes. "It's kind of like your place was bombed and the police show up, then the ambulance shows up, then the army, and then the construction workers," Traber explains.

But it's not a perfect system. If your body is repeatedly repairing damage done by a constant stream of bomblike free radicals, eventually your cells will show the cumulative wear and tear of all that destruction, like an old beat-up car that's been fixed and repainted multiple times. Over time, this effect builds up and contributes to aging. Studies have shown that oxidative stress plays a role in many facets of aging, including wrinkles, graying hair, and cancer.

> "Eventually your cells will show the cumulative wear and tear of all that destruction, like an old beat-up car that's been fixed and repainted multiple times."

"There is an increased accumulation of free radical damage as you grow older, that's irrefutable," says Dr. Jeffrey B. Blumburg, director of the Antioxidants Research Laboratory at the Jean Mayer USDA Human Nutrition Research Center on Aging at Tufts University. "You can see biomarkers of that—accumulations of free radical damage—particularly in long-lived cells like neurons in the brain."

Oxidative stress also produces a vicious cycle of more oxidative stress. Take the mitochondria, for example. As the engine that creates free radicals, it's often the first part of the cell to be damaged by free radicals as they flail around. That damage is quickly repaired, but over many years, the mitochondria get worn down by this constant assault, making them less efficient. When they're less efficient, they produce even more free radicals, which cause even more damage, and so on.

The exact role of radicals and oxidative stress in aging is still not fully understood. One reason is because scientists also know that free radicals perform some beneficial functions. They have long been known as a key component in certain immune responses, for example. British scientists recently found that the presence of free radicals jumps markedly in tadpoles if their tails are cut off—and stays elevated while the tail regenerates. When researchers greatly limited a tadpole's free radical production, either through antioxidants or genetic manipulation, its tail failed to grow back.

What the body appears to need, then, is a balance of radicals and antioxidants. Yet a wide variety of dietary and lifestyle factors can get this balance way out of whack. Smoking is a huge creator of radicals in your cells. So is overeating or eating the wrong foods; sun exposure; exercising too intensively; and exposure to chemicals. The more oxidative stress your body experiences, the more out of balance your system becomes and the more damage is inflicted on your cells.

You'll find more about this critically important facet of metabolism, and how to regulate it, later in the book.

Cell Surrender

The free radicals generated by metabolism also damage the DNA in your cells, which causes yet another set of problems. The instructions for cell replication are coded into the DNA inside a cell's nucleus. When that's damaged by oxidative stress, it can cause mutations or damage in subsequent cells, which can then malfunction, stop replicating, or die. That might sound like a terrible outcome, but cell death is actually part of life.

In the typical adult, *billions* of cells die every day, and you want it that way. A person whose cells never died through natural, pre-programmed means would succumb to cancer at an early age. The body's ability to make its own cells self-destruct provides critical protection against cancer, a disease whose hallmark is unchecked cell growth. When cancer cells grow without stopping, they also destroy healthy tissue and organs.

Programmed cell death (PCD) also helps get rid of older, damaged cells so new ones, with peak abilities, can take their place. If a cell's function declines to a certain point—from oxidative stress, for example—a special enzyme triggers an irreversible process of cell suicide, and it disintegrates. PCD even plays a role in making people look the way they do. For example, it's the process that causes the fleshy webbing between a developing baby's fingers and toes to disintegrate so the baby is born with fingers and toes instead of webbed hands and feet.

Not all cells go through these concrete stages of life and death, however. There's an in-between stage in which a cell no longer has the ability to divide, but it isn't dead either. This stage, called *senescence,* is being widely linked to aging.

When you're young, most cells in your body divide about 50 to 70 times before they die or stop replicating. It's a process that's essential to generate new bone, blood, or tissue when needed. Then, after that maximum number of divisions has been reached, cells go into a resting phase, called senescence. Scientists believe this is a natural defense against cancer because it limits the cells' ability to become cancerous and continue dividing indefinitely. But it's not foolproof. Without the ability to replicate or die, senescent cells are at risk of functioning abnormally, which can also cause them to become cancerous.

"The body's ability to make its own cells self-destruct offers critical protection against cancer, a disease whose hallmark is unchecked cell growth."

What's more, senescent cells emit proteins that cause inflammation in the surrounding tissue. Some scientists think these proteins are a cell's attempt to be protective: by summoning your immune system to the region and clearing out senescent cells before they become a problem.

In younger, healthy people, the immune system efficiently clears out any senescent cells. But there aren't that many senescent cells in younger people's bodies to begin with, because fewer cells have reached their division limits. The older you get, though, the more senescent cells you have, not only because more cells have reached the end of their replication abilities, but also because older peoples' immune systems aren't as efficient.

The result is you get an accumulation of senescent cells as you age, and these have been linked to cell abnormalities such as cancer, but also to a general reduction in the appearance and function of normal tissue, leading to many conditions commonly associated with aging, such as heart disease.

How much of aging is the result of cell senescence? That's not clear, but a groundbreaking study done at the Mayo Clinic and published in the journal *Nature* in November 2011 suggests a strong link. In the experiment, researchers managed to virtually halt aging in a group of mice just by cleaning out all their senescent cells with genetically targeted drugs. Without those inactive cells, the mice stayed youthful and vigorous, with firm tissue, plenty of energy, and healthy hair. This study offers tantalizing evidence that senescence could be a linchpin in the aging process. As you would expect, a flood of research on cell senescence has begun.

> "Without those inactive cells, the mice stayed youthful and vigorous, with firm tissue, plenty of energy, and healthy hair. This study offers tantalizing evidence that senescence could be a linchpin in the aging process."

Ironically, both senescence and PCD help prevent cancer in younger people, yet can contribute to it in older people. Throughout evolution, this hasn't created much of an issue because, until very recently, the human life expectancy was so low. For tens of thousands of years, most humans lived to only about 25 or 30 years old, dying early of disease, infection, or starvation long before their bodies got the chance to age. But with advances in sanitation, medicine, and nutrition pushing our lifespans into the 70s and beyond, we are seeing the downside of some of the systems employed by evolution to protect us when we're young and fertile.

Of course, you're still thinking about those mice—and what you can do to get your hands on those drugs that made them stay young and healthy! Unfortunately, that's a long way off: the mice were genetically altered to respond to the drugs they were given. But that doesn't mean senescence is insurmountable. A growing body of evidence suggests that certain dietary factors can influence how much your cells senesce. One study, for example, published in 2011 in the journal *Age,* found that consuming a traditional Mediterranean diet, which includes a lot of olive oil, fish, legumes, fruits, and vegetables, reduced the level of cellular senescence in elderly subjects. (You learn more about this later in the book.)

Trimming Telomeres

One of the great developments in aging research in recent years is the discovery of telomeres, which are like protective caps on the ends of chromosomes, the double strands of DNA inside the nucleus of a cell. Telomeres are often compared to aglets, the little plastic tips that keep the ends of shoelaces from unraveling.

Telomeres are necessary because every time a cell divides, the strands of DNA inside the new cell get a tiny bit shorter. Before a cell can divide, the original DNA must first be duplicated, so there's a copy for the mother cell and a copy for the subsequent cell. But the little mechanism inside your cells that makes this DNA copy is actually attached to the end of it, sort of like a pastry bag squeezing out icing. So when it gets down to the very end of the DNA strand, the little pastry bag is in the way so it can't replicate the very tip of the chain.

Luckily, the last 8,000 or so pairs of amino acids at the ends of your DNA strands (which are 150 million pairs long!) are different from the rest of the DNA strand. They do not contain any actual genetic information, so losing a portion of this section won't cause any genetic mutations to be passed on to the subsequent cell. This differentiated portion of the DNA chain is the telomere. Each time the cell divides, the telomeres get shorter and shorter. Once they get too short to trim again without damaging the actual genetic code, the cell becomes senescent.

Telomere length can be a good barometer of aging. Older individuals typically have shorter telomeres, which makes sense because their cells have divided more times through their lives. But that's not the whole story. Two people who are the same age can have telomeres of very different lengths, suggesting that some people preserve telomere length better than others.

> "Two people who are the same age can have telomeres of very different lengths, suggesting that some people preserve telomere length better than others."

A group of scientists won the Nobel Prize for Medicine in 2009 for their discovery of telomeres, as well as an enzyme, called telomerase, that can lengthen telomeres. Telomerase is found abundantly in some cells, such as human eggs and sperm, which have telomeres that never shorten. But it's also found in cancer cells, where the enzyme allows for unending cell division.

So what accounts for the longer telomeres in some people? Numerous studies are looking into factors that influence the length of telomeres. Stress appears to play an adverse role, as indicated by one study that showed that mothers of chronically ill children have shorter telomeres. It makes sense, then, that stress-reduction behaviors, such as meditation and exercise, have been shown to increase the body's natural production of telomerase and lengthen telomeres. Other diet and lifestyle changes are also being studied for their impact on telomere length, with promising results.

Would you like to know how long your telomeres are? Several start-up companies want to make it easy for you to get your telomeres measured so you can have a concrete measurement of your aging progression. On one hand, having this information could be a little alarming. On the other, it would provide a great incentive to make behavioral and lifestyle changes that are known to slow or reverse the process of telomere shortening.

Indeed, telomeres may play an important role in keeping younger people healthy. In a study published in February 2013 in the *Journal of the American Medical Association,* a team of researchers from Carnegie Mellon University exposed 152 individuals ages 18 to 55 to a common cold virus. The subjects with shorter immune-cell telomeres experienced greater rates of actual infection with the virus.

Protein Origami

Proteins are essential to life: they play a role in virtually every function of your cells, including metabolism; the cycle of a cell's life; immunity; and even structural elements outside of your cells, such as collagen. Made of chains of amino acids, proteins can provide transportation for vitamins and other molecules, binding to them to carry them around, or protection, capturing rogue elements in your cells and neutralizing them. Many hormones are proteins, too, including insulin, which controls your blood-sugar concentration, and oxytocin, which stimulates a woman's body to go into contractions during childbirth. Proteins can act alone or in connection with other proteins. In short, they are incredibly important and highly complex. And you have tens of thousands of them in your body!

Now researchers are discovering that how proteins behave inside and outside your cells can affect the way you age. Dr. Steven Austad, the scientist working with clams at the University of Texas, is researching the way these complex molecules are structured and how those structures affect the protein's behavior.

"Proteins in your body either form structures, or they help chemical reactions," Austad explains. "To do that they're folded up in these intricate ways like origami. But as they get older they start to lose the precise folding they used to have."

And this is where problems can arise. When proteins are folded correctly into their specific three-dimensional forms, they are stable and can maintain their physical properties. For example, a protein that's very tightly wound might be especially resistant to interacting with other molecules. But if that same protein unfolds slightly, or misfolds during formation, its exposed surface might accidentally bind to other molecules, or to another protein, which can keep it from performing the job it was intended for.

These damaged proteins are implicated in numerous age-related diseases, especially in the brain. In Alzheimer's disease, for example, proteins misfold and bind to each other, forming plaques in the brain that gradually destroy the brain's ability to function properly. Because protein damage increases as you age, these kinds of diseases tend to appear later in life.

In the field of aging, Austad is what's known as a comparative biologist, which means he looks at how other species do something better than we humans do and tries to figure out how they do it. "What we think, and what we have quite a bit of evidence for, is that the [species] that are best at maintaining their protein folding are the ones that live the longest," he says.

Take, for example, that 500-year-old clam with the heart that was beating even before Shakespeare. In a decidedly unpoetic experiment, Austad's team essentially chopped up one of these clams and made a kind of clam serum. To that serum, the researchers added the kinds of proteins found in Alzheimer's that normally would clump together. But in the clam serum, those same proteins did not clump together. What Austad wants to know now is "whether they have some sort of substance that is really good at keeping proteins folded."

Other researchers have studied the precise protein folding found in the cells of the naked mole rat, a rodent so unbelievably ugly it's actually cute. Naked mole rats are a favorite of aging researchers because they're the world's longest-lived rodents: they live to be 30 or 40 years old and exhibit few of the typical age-related diseases, such as heart disease, diabetes, and cancer. Yet those diseases do afflict the naked mole rat's furry cousins, mice, which live to just 3 or 4 years.

But the naked mole rat, even if it stays remarkably healthy through much of its life, is otherwise not so enviable: they are buck-toothed, almost blind, cold-blooded, and hairless, and they eat their own excrement. Not exactly the life you'd pick. Roughly the same size as mice, they live in complex, oxygen-starved, underground colonies with a social structure reminiscent of ants or bees. Plenty of researchers are looking at what these rodents have going for them that allows them to live so long and so well—indeed, cancer has never been detected in a naked mole rat. Precise protein folding is one definite possibility. A study published in 2009 in the *Proceedings of the National Academy of Sciences* found that naked mole rats have "remarkable resistance to protein unfolding."

An interesting fact about naked mole rats is that they show high levels of oxidative stress in their cells, yet it doesn't seem to damage their proteins the way oxidative stress does in mice—or even people. Like Austad's clam, they may have a special enzyme or system that keeps their proteins perfectly folded, but that's still unclear.

> "Cancer has never been detected in a naked mole rat."

Researchers are just beginning to identify some of the factors that lead to protein misfolding in people and what mechanisms help them fold correctly. Several studies have found that proteins can misfold when they're damaged by oxidative stress or when DNA is damaged by oxidative stress. That's because it's the genes in your DNA that are responsible for creating the proteins in your body, so if the DNA is damaged, it can create malfunctioning proteins. The human body also has a complex network of signals and systems that help proteins fold correctly, assisted by other proteins called chaperones, but those also can be damaged by environmental factors. This isn't well understood, but it could be one reason certain diet and lifestyle factors—such as a diet high in omega-3 fatty acids—seem to protect people from diseases like Alzheimer's that feature malformed proteins.

Genetic Influences

Scientists have plenty of evidence that aging can be influenced by lifestyle and behavior, but obviously genes also play a clear role in a person's health and, especially, longevity.

Research has identified many genes that might control a person's predisposition to develop a particular age-related health problem—or not. For example, people with certain versions of a gene involved in metabolizing fats and carbohydrates are at greater risk of developing cardiovascular disease. Scientists also have identified variants of genes that predispose people to develop Alzheimer's and variants that seem to protect them from cognitive decline.

But assessing all the genetic variables that lead to a healthier, longer life borders on the impossible. The human genome is made up of about 20,000 to 25,000 genes and 3 billion base pairs of amino acids. Many hundreds, or even thousands, of them likely play a role in aging.

There was a watershed moment in the field of genetics and aging more than a decade ago, when scientists discovered that altering one particular gene in the roundworm caused it to live twice as long—and not just twice as long by extending its old age, but twice as long with the health and vitality of a younger worm. The gene in question was involved in the regulation of and response to insulin, a critical hormone in metabolism. In humans, one group of researchers identified at least 30 genes involved in just that one insulin-regulating process.

> "Scientists discovered that altering one particular gene in the roundworm caused it to live twice as long ... with the health and vitality of a younger worm."

But could these genes influence aging in humans? How would you know? To learn more, researchers looked for those 30 genes in very elderly women from Sardinia, an Italian island where the population is relatively homogeneous, making it a useful place to do genetic research. Among the 30 genes, they found one that was expressed in most of the elderly women in the study. The results suggest that there is a genetic component to aging—but they also illuminate how difficult it is to figure out what role each gene might play.

Where genes really seem to play an enormous role is in determining extreme longevity. The role of genetics is obvious in families that include multiple long-lived individuals. In fact, extreme longevity tends to cluster in families; it's not unusual to find a healthy person in his or her 90s—or older!—who also has a sibling in the same age range, or who had a parent who lived that long. These people seem to share some lucky genetic signaling, although no one has figured out exactly what that is. A study published in early 2012 in the online journal *PLoS One,* for example, looked at the genes of 800 centenarians and found that 90 percent of them had groupings of 26 particular genes known to be related to aging. It's clear those genes are involved, but it's a lot more complicated to figure out the relationship than if it were just one or two genes.

Promising research on longevity has been conducted by Dr. Nir Barzilai at the Albert Einstein College of Medicine in New York. Dr. Barzilai has found remarkable evidence for the influence of genetics on exceptionally long-lived individuals through his LonGenity research program, which is studying a group of about 500 centenarians and 700 of their offspring, ages 60 to 85. His research clearly shows that longevity can be inherited and is very strongly associated with high levels of "good" (HDL) cholesterol and low "bad" (LDL) cholesterol.

But the role of genetics is much less clear in typical aging and all its associated illnesses, including diabetes, cancer, and heart disease. Some of the most widely quoted research in the field comes from Scandinavian studies of twins. Sweden, for example, has a registry of 70,000 pairs of twins born in the country between 1886 and 1990, giving scientists a rich resource for studying the lifestyle and genetic influences on twins. From this database, researchers have been able to follow identical twins who were separated as children and raised apart, either in different households or families. Because identical twins have all the same genes, this research made it possible to look at which factors of aging are the result of lifestyle or behavior and which are the result of their shared genetics. Researchers found decreasing genetic influence throughout the lives of those identical twins raised separately.

In some cases, the genetic influence on certain diseases was found to be as low as 8 or 9 percent, but the study found that if one twin ate poorly and exercised little, while the other twin grew up to live a healthier, active lifestyle, their health outcomes in middle age and old age were starkly different. What's more, even twins who shared a genetic predisposition to get a particular age-related condition did not necessarily develop that condition at the same time if the two individuals had markedly different lifestyles. In other words, the likelihood of developing age-related diseases was found to be highly dependent on environmental factors, especially later in life.

Results like this have made the case—now widely accepted by scientists—that even in the general population, genes are like a hand of cards you are dealt: you have to play the game right to win. You can have a lousy set of cards but still come from behind and score big. Or if you look like a winner in the beginning but are careless about your next move, you can lose it all.

> "Genes are like a hand of cards you are dealt: you have to play the game right to win."

Only a small subset of people have the genetics that allow them to live to be super-old. Everyone else lives by the normal rules of aging: you have to make an effort to age well.

Individuals who live to be extremely old are a select group who have avoided the many chronic health problems that usually characterize old age. Many of them didn't necessarily follow good dietary or lifestyle choices, yet they managed to live longer than any actuarial table would predict. These special people make up a different kind of "1 percent."

In the 2010 U.S. Census, just 1.5 percent of the population was age 85 and older, and just a fraction of 1 percent of Americans live to be 100 or older. To put this in perspective, in a packed stadium of 25,000 sports fans, maybe 10 people will reach the century mark. Those who live that long, science suggests, won the genetic lottery; something in their genes protects them from the usual declines and diseases of aging.

But the vast majority of people—that is, everyone else in the stadium—do not have that special mix of genes. They are stuck with the fact that *what they do* is going to largely determine how they fare in the coming years. As Austad, the comparative biologist from the University of Texas, put it: "If you want to live to be a healthy 80-year-old, you need to eat right and get the right amount of exercise. If you want to live to be a healthy 100-year-old, you need to have the right parents."

You Control Your Genes

That genes are only somewhat involved in the typical aging process is on display nowhere more than in studies of identical twins raised separately. In these cases, even the genes that supposedly determine our risk for heart disease and Alzheimer's are not clearly in control.

But if not genes, then what is in control?

You are, because your genes actually change over the years.

Throughout your lifetime, environmental factors such as diet and stress cause subtle variations to the outer structure of your genes, which is called the *epigenome*. These changes can determine how much of an influence a particular gene has in determining your health, personality, lifespan, and more. They can even get passed on to the next generation.

This outer layer of instructions surrounding your genes acts like multiple on and off switches for your DNA. Epigenetic changes are fundamental to the normal development of an embryo; it is epigenetic switches that make cells become one thing or another, such as a liver cell or a brain cell, during development.

Although this field is just emerging and scientists need to do a lot more research to understand the causes and effects of epigenetics, the discoveries are rewriting a lot of the old thinking about nature versus nurture.

Here's how epigenetic changes work: your DNA is made of two long strands of genes (which are sequences of nucleic acids) that are wound together in a three-dimensional shape. But over time, little pieces of molecular baggage called *methyl groups* can attach themselves to specific genes on your DNA, causing those genes to be expressed differently.

Let's look, for example, at a woman with a gene that puts her at higher risk of getting breast cancer. If a methyl group attaches to that gene and suppresses its function, her risk of getting breast cancer is reduced to the same level as a woman who doesn't have that breast cancer gene. This methylation is sort of like permanent makeup for your genes.

Scientists are identifying numerous factors that appear to influence methylation, including chronic stress, environmental chemicals, or even the food you eat. Although each person has only one genome, with the same sequence of genes on all the copies of his or her DNA, continual methylation throughout life means a person can have multiple epigenomes. That's because the DNA in different kinds of cells and tissues develop different epigenetic markers through the years, influencing the behavior and health of just those cells or tissues.

The power of this process became a sensation about 10 years ago when researchers did an experiment on mutant mice. The species of mouse used would normally be brown and thin, but these mice had one mutated gene that made their fur yellow and caused them to overeat uncontrollably, making them obese and prone to diabetes. Before the mice got pregnant, and until their pups were weaned, researchers fed the female mice a diet with large quantities of vitamins that are known to produce methyl groups in the body, including B_{12}, folic acid, and choline. Rather than being born yellow and becoming fat, all the babies were born brown and stayed thin. The baby mice had in fact inherited the mutated gene that causes obesity and yellow fur, but it had been deactivated by a methyl group from the mother's diet. What the mother ate, before and during pregnancy, protected her babies from a genetic mutation.

Changes to the epigenome are thought to have developed as an evolutionary benefit that created spontaneous genetic variation in an otherwise homogeneous group, thereby enhancing the group's chances of survival. It also allowed people to adjust, even across generations, when environmental influences suddenly changed. Experiments in lab animals, for example, have demonstrated that if a mother is undernourished during pregnancy, her babies are likely to be born with various traits that help them survive in an environment with little food. Baboon mothers fed a poor, nutrient-deficient diet, for

"What the mother ate, before and during pregnancy, protected her babies from a genetic mutation."

example, gave birth to babies whose livers churned out glucose—a helpful characteristic if there was little food to eat.

The epigenetic effects we pass onto our children begin to accumulate well before pregnancy, too. Other studies have found that people who dramatically overate as children later had kids and even grandkids with shortened lifespans. Men who began smoking before puberty had sons who lived shorter lives, as well.

Epigenetic changes continue throughout life, a phenomenon known as *epigenetic drift*. If you've ever known a pair of identical twins, you know that they tend to look almost indistinguishable as youngsters, but they begin to develop slightly different appearances, and even different levels of health, as they get older. Those factors are the result of modifications to their epigenomes, which are undergoing constant methylation throughout life. The addition of these methyl groups to their genetic structure causes some genes to be overexpressed and others to be underexpressed. Some studies have clearly pointed to certain environmental factors that can influence specific genes, but the research into this kind of cause and effect is really just beginning.

Some scientists have found that certain foods can influence positive epigenetic effects. Dr. Trygve O. Tollefsbol, a molecular biologist at the University of Alabama, studies epigenetic influences on cancer and aging. He believes epigenetic influences are a new frontier in the effort to stay healthy and live a longer life.

Tollefsbol's lab has identified several regular foods, such as broccoli and green tea, that suppress cancer in animals through this epigenomic effect. A lot more needs to be learned, and the compounds need to be studied in humans to have concrete scientific proof. But Tollefsbol is convinced—as are other scientists working on similar projects—that identifying the epigenetic effects of different foods and behaviors could dramatically improve the way we age. It would also, Tollefsbol hopes, encourage

"Identifying the epigenetic effects of different foods and behaviors could dramatically improve the way we age."

an attitude change about aging, shifting the emphasis from medical treatment of age-related conditions to prevention throughout life. He has been credited with coining the term *epigenetics diet,* but so far that diet is pretty narrow, even if its effects are very impressive.

"Things like this can affect millions of people," Tollefsbol says. "What I'm talking about is the millions of us who want to prevent getting cancer in the first place, or to extend our longevity. The earlier in life we can implement this, even by our mothers' consuming some of these compounds, then the better."

Aging and Smoking

If you care about the way you're going to age, there's no way around this statement:

> *Almost nothing will age you more, and faster, than smoking.*

It's well known that smoking dramatically increases a person's risk of getting cancer, but even more fundamentally, it ages you in almost every way. Smoking constricts blood vessels, robbing cells of needed oxygen and nutrients. It causes extreme levels of oxidative stress inside cells, damaging DNA—as well as the mechanisms designed to fix that DNA once it's been harmed. The toxins in cigarette smoke pass through cell membranes and, once inside, overwhelm the body's cell-cleaning mechanisms, meaning they can't clean up other harmful compounds. Smoking even reduces the levels of some vitamins in the bloodstream.

These and other damaging effects of smoking promote heart disease, lung problems, cancer, cognitive decline, cataracts, and many other systemic health problems usually associated with advanced age. It also causes premature wrinkling of the skin, thinning of the hair, brittle nails, and other cosmetic signs of aging.

Here are some recent scientific studies highlighting other ways smoking is harmful:

A study conducted by Severine Sabia at the University College of London and published in 2012 showed that middle-aged men who smoked had an increased rate of cognitive decline, measured in four areas: memory, vocabulary, executive function, and global function.

A study conducted by J. Edwin Blalock at the University of Alabama, Birmingham, published in 2010 showed that cigarette smoke blocks a key enzyme the body uses to regulate its response to inflammation.

A study by Toru Nyunoya at the University of Iowa in 2009 found that smoking damages a key protein that protects cells from cancer and aging. It's the same protein that's defective in individuals with Werner's Syndrome, a rare disease that causes rapid, premature aging, beginning at puberty, resulting in early death.

About 20 percent of U.S. adults smoke. If you are a smoker, you have every reason to quit, and many of the conditions caused by smoking begin receding as soon as you stop. When you're young and seem healthy enough, it's easy to think you'll be one of the lucky ones who escape lung cancer, emphysema, heart disease, dementia, or any of the other conditions linked to smoking, but it's a huge gamble, and you're betting with your life.

Empowered Aging

If there's one thing this quick lesson in the science of aging should have conveyed, it's that there is every reason to be optimistic about growing older because so much of it is within your control. Most of the processes scientists have identified as playing a major role in aging at the cellular level—including oxidative stress, senescence and cell death, telomere shortening, damaged proteins, and epigenetics— have been shown in studies to be influenced by dietary and lifestyle factors. It's why people who lead healthy lives with good nutrition and solid health habits, like my husband, age better.

Which gets us back to the original question at the beginning of this chapter: how do you envision yourself in old age? When asked this question, participants in the Baltimore Longitudinal Study on Aging who gave a positive, upbeat assessment of where they'd be 20, 30, 40 years later were much more likely to have aged well after all those years had passed. People who were negative or pessimistic about old age, meanwhile, tended to age that way, too.

It's one of the many intriguing pieces of evidence that certain attitudes, such as openness to change, happiness, and optimism, are contributing factors in how people age. Exactly why or how is unclear, but it's reason enough to try to change your perceptions about aging—and the best way to do that is to know that you are doing something about it. Rather than worry about aging or avoid thinking about it, just grab the reins and start pulling.

Because here's what really matters: you don't have to make huge changes to your life to affect the way you age. You can tweak your routine bit by bit over time and still make a huge difference in what your life will be like 5, 10, or 20 years from now. When you're trying to influence the way you age, one thing you *do* have is time.

Just follow the science. It's like a cheat-sheet for staying young.

Part 2

The Nutrition Solution

Nutrition Now, Aging Later

There is no cure for aging, but there *are* ways to slow it down, and one of the best is through nutrition. As the science of aging becomes clearer, and the impact of diet is better understood, more and more scientists are starting to see the food we eat as the key to aging well.

Dr. Luigi Ferrucci of the National Institute on Aging says scientists "are barely scratching the surface" when it comes to the causes of aging. But he is convinced that even after whatever discoveries lie ahead, and whatever drugs are created as a result of those discoveries, the ultimate conclusion will remain quite simple. "Nutrition is going to be one of the most important aspects to modulate aging—more than the interventions we have," he says.

Yet far too few Americans know that such an easy solution can keep many of the symptoms of aging at bay. People know that eating better will make them healthier, or thinner, but few people equate eating with aging.

Science, however, is proving how inextricably linked they are. Eating too much and eating the wrong things doesn't just lead to overt health problems, such as obesity, dementia, diabetes, and heart disease. It also affects us at the cellular level, impacting all those aging factors discussed in the previous chapter, such as oxidative stress, the length of your telomeres, and the signals of your epigenome.

Yet what most Americans eat suggests they don't really understand what a big difference their diet makes to their health today and in the future. It affects how they feel, how they'll age, and even their risk for developing diseases such as cancer and Alzheimer's.

According to the U.S. Department of Agriculture, the typical American woman age 31 to 50 consumes just 14 grams fiber a day, when the recommended adequate intake is 25 grams. She eats 230 grams carbohydrates a day—a whopping 100 more than is recommended. And she gets about 70 grams protein daily, when she only needs 46.

Clock-Cheater Tip

A great first step to improving your diet is to find out what you *should* be eating in terms of nutrients. Go to the USDA's Food and Nutrition Information Center website at fnic.nal.usda.gov/dietary-guidance for excellent resources.

The typical man in the same age group is no better: he eats a little more than 100 grams protein a day, but needs only 56. He eats well more than twice the 130 grams carbohydrates he should in a day, but he falls far short on fiber, eating only 18 grams when 38 grams is considered adequate.

The result of such careless consumption is that nearly 36 percent of the U.S. population is obese, according to the Centers for Disease Control. And only 25 percent eats the recommended five servings of fruits and vegetables a day. Together, these statistics point to a coming tidal wave of illness, disease, premature aging, and early death.

But who wants to end up that way? No one. So why the disconnect?

Based on my reporting, and after watching my husband's transformation, I believe there are three main problems keeping Americans from eating in a way that will help them live a longer, healthier life. They are all related, and they can all be overcome simply by taking a different approach:

Problem 1: It's hard for people to change what they eat.

Solution: Let's face it, no one wants to give up the tasty foods they love, even if those foods are unhealthy. Plus, your body gets used to eating a certain way, making it even harder to change your habits. The way around this is to make changes to your diet very slowly, even so slowly they're almost unnoticeable. If you let good habits develop over time—even years—you eventually won't *want* to eat any (or as many) unhealthy foods.

Problem 2: People don't think small changes make a difference.

Solution: Small changes don't show results in a week or two, so people don't feel motivated to stick with them. But by understanding the science of aging, and how those small changes are working *at the cellular level,* they become more meaningful and easier to stick with.

Problem 3: People don't want to take months or years to improve their health and looks.

Solution: When it comes to self-improvement, people want immediate results. They want to look better *now,* or at least next week or next month. But healthy aging should be a separate goal; if you also want to live longer and stay in better health for years to come, decide to make small changes for that reason. You *will* end up looking and feeling better, but it will take a while.

Just as there are many factors that cause aging, there are many things you can do to turn it back. But nutrition is the key—the low-hanging fruit, if you will. All it takes is a slight attitude adjustment: you must accept that it doesn't matter if it takes months or years to look and feel better, as long as you get there, one way or another. The only sure thing is that if you do nothing, you definitely won't get anywhere!

> "Nutrition is the key—the low-hanging fruit."

Small Changes, Big Difference

If you approach aging the right way, you'll feel good about it right away. By starting with minor changes now, you immediately put yourself on the path to a healthier you for years to come. Of course, that doesn't mean you can eat one less Snickers bar a week and call it a day.

The reward is proportional, so the healthier your diet is today, the greater the benefit will be in future years. The beauty of eating for aging is that any healthy changes you make, if you stick with them, become magnified over the years. And once you've made one healthy lifestyle change, however small, it tends to lead to others—and it gets easier.

My husband's experience has borne out the effectiveness of that strategy. This is a man who coined the term "travel hungry," for eating whatever looked good when you're on vacation, hungry or not. But without actively trying to lose weight or change his diet, the small tweaks Jim began to make years ago eventually added up to real change, and everything else followed. Today he looks better and feels better than he ever could have imagined at age 64—and now I would have to sedate him to get him to eat a Cinnabon in an airport terminal.

The success of Jim's approach was in not focusing on his weight next week or next month, but on his health next *year* and next *decade*. Because he had children late in life—we had our first child when he was 50!—he had to think this way. He wants to be there to see them grow up and to provide for them.

This difference in perspective is not only critical, it's revolutionary.

Think of it like this: if you are planning at all for your financial future, whether it's retirement or college tuition or anything else, think about saving for your future health the same way by improving your nutrition, bit by bit. If you don't manage to "save" for 1 week or 1 month, it doesn't matter in the long term, as long as you start up again. It's the cumulative effect of saving—saving your health—that makes a difference.

Clock-Cheater Tip

Make a plan for retirement—a health plan. If you've thought about how much money you'll need when you retire, do the same for your health: set goals for how healthy you want to be. Is your goal to be able to play golf? Then you want to be sure you stay physically fit. Do you want to travel? Then you want to do everything you can to keep your brain sharp. Now work backward: what will you need to do between now and then to reach those goals? This exercise helps you view your health as a long-term effort—just like bank savings.

For this approach to work for you, you need to do two things:

Forget about your history with food, your weight, or your poor choices, and try something new. Shift your focus from how you feel about yourself today, and think instead about how you want to feel in the future. That doesn't mean you shouldn't worry about what's going on now. It simply means that the things you do toward the goal of aging well may have no impact on how you look and feel now. They will eventually, but it will take time.

Learn the science about what affects aging. This is fundamental, because if you make a small change to your diet or lifestyle and you barely notice the change to your weight or skin or energy level, you're likely to say what anyone in your situation would: "Okaaaay, *this* isn't working." But if you know the science, you'll know it *is* working, whether you see the difference today or not. You won't see it like money accumulating in a bank account, but you'll know that what you're doing is doing good. That's the best way to make yourself stick with it. (So if you haven't read the previous chapter about the science of aging, you should go back and read it now!)

Mind the Message

Our bodies were designed over tens of thousands of years to be the perfect digestion machines for the foods available to us at that time. For millennia, that meant a largely plant-based diet with the occasional, much-appreciated influx of animal protein from a hunt. Thousands of years ago, of course, the average humans didn't live very long, for other reasons. But our bodies are still built to need the same vital kinds of nutrition that we have consumed over thousands of years.

Clock-Cheater Tip

Don't just think about whether your food is caloric or fatty or nutritious. Think about whether it's the kind of food ancient humans would have had available. That's the kind of food your body was designed to eat—fresh, even raw, and unprocessed. The more food you eat that doesn't pass that simple test, the more your body ages on the inside.

By eating the foods our bodies were designed to eat, it's like putting the right gasoline in your car—which most people do. Who wants to invest in a car and then have it start knocking and rattling?

Eating the right food sounds simple enough. I always considered myself a relatively healthy eater, so when I started investigating this subject, I wasn't expecting any surprises. But the more I learned about the factors that influence aging, the more I realized that the healthiest part of my eating habits was that I didn't *over*eat. That's important, for sure, but I never knew how clueless I was about *what* to eat until I started looking at my husband's habits.

Although the health and fitness industry touts good-for-you foods, and the government has done a good job of simplifying its nutrition recommendations so they're easier to understand, it's still hard to get the right messages about food. Take the recent $1 summer drink promotion at McDonald's: a 32-ounce Coca-Cola, with its 350 calories and 86 grams of sugar (20 teaspoons!), for just $1—less than the cost of a simple bottle of water. A drink with 20 teaspoons sugar and no nutrition clearly is not the right fuel for your body.

> "I never knew how clueless I was about *what* to eat until I started looking at my husband's habits."

When we make bad choices, we can justify our decisions by hiding behind the stories of people who took great care of themselves but were struck down young—like Jim Fixx, the famous running and fitness enthusiast who dropped dead of a heart attack in 1984 at age 52. Or we can hope to be one of the lucky ones who breeze through life despite horrifying habits, like my Great Aunt Eppie.

When I was growing up, Eppie smoked a pack of unfiltered Pall Mall cigarettes a day, fried her (white) bread in sausage grease, and always kept a bottle of Kentucky Gentleman bourbon on the floor next to her chair at the kitchen table. She sat there for much of the day, nattering and bickering with her sister (my grandmother) and obsessively reading the stock tables of the *Winston-Salem Courier-Journal* with a magnifying glass. For these vices, she died at age 92 after a brief illness.

But in studying the Eppies and Jim Fixxes of the world—whose genetics undoubtedly played a crucial role in their unusually long and short lifespans, respectively—here's what scientists have figured out: the vast majority of Americans live and grow old in the large middle ground between these two extremes. And it's this group of "everyone else" who can actually make a difference in how they age by eating a healthier diet.

Nothing is a guarantee, and science is not about promises. There are always going to be some people who simply have an unlucky set of genes and will get sick when they're far too young no matter what they do. But science can usually tell us what works most of the time for most of the people. And the vast majority of healthy people can greatly influence how much energy they will have, how healthy they will be, and how youthful they will remain in the years to come.

Save Your Cells

Your health in the second half of your life is partly determined by your genes, whether you ate well as a child, and even by whether your mother ate well as a child (the epigenetic effect). But the over-whelming evidence is that your diet and lifestyle have the biggest influence on you from middle age and beyond. If you've always eaten poorly and finally decide to eat better starting at age 40 or 50—good milestones to make changes!—you can make a big difference, almost right away, in your health, your looks, and your vitality.

One of my favorite studies to show this effect was done by researchers at the Medical University of South Carolina and published in 2007 in *The American Journal of Medicine*. It followed more than 15,000 subjects ages 45 to 64 for 10 years. At the outset, few of the participants lived what the study authors called a "healthy lifestyle," which they defined as eating at least five daily servings of fruits and vegetables, not smoking, not being obese, and getting regular exercise. Six years later, another small portion of the group (slightly less than 10 percent) had *adopted* those healthy habits. The study followed them for another 4 years and found these new adopters showed significant improvements in health, including halving their rate of cardiovascular events and overall mortality than the subjects who did not change their habits.

The study's conclusion? "People who newly adopt a healthy life-style in middle age experience a prompt benefit of lower rates of cardiovascular disease and mortality."

What I love about this study is that it tracked participants who had made healthy changes at any point over those 6 years! They started out in the unhealthy category, but 6 years later, they were living a healthier lifestyle. That time frame seems impossibly long in the quick-fix, weight-loss-focused world we live in. What self-respecting diet would come with the promise to "look slimmer in 6 years"? No one would go on a diet like that! But what if you knew the payoff after 6 years was that you get to live longer? The message of this study is clear: even if you take 6 years to slowly change your habits into healthier ones, the benefits rack up quickly.

The study published in 2011 in the journal *Age,* that looked at the impact of the Mediterranean diet on aging, is another great example. In this study out of Spain, elderly subjects were divided into three groups and fed three different diets for 4 weeks. One group received a diet high in saturated fats; one group ate a low-fat, high-carbohydrate diet; and the third ate a classic Mediterranean diet, including fruits, vegetables, fish, and healthy fats such as olive oil. After just a month, the researchers studied cells from the subject's vascular system. Compared with the other two groups and to the baseline measurements at the start of the study, the group that ate a Mediterranean diet showed a lower level of cellular senescence and cell death and fewer cells with shortening telomeres. In other words, what they ate had slowed down the aging process.

"What self-respecting diet would come with the promise to 'look slimmer in 6 years?' No one would go on a diet like that! But what if you knew the payoff after 6 years was that you get to live longer?"

Clock-Cheater Tip

Easily eat more Mediterranean by using olive oil, a healthy fat, in place of butter for cooking. You can use a pastry brush to spread it on sandwich bread instead of using mayonnaise.

In a recent study, Spanish researchers divided more than 7,000 individuals age 55 to 80 into three groups: one following a Mediterranean diet supplemented with extra-virgin olive oil, one following a Mediterranean diet supplemented with mixed nuts, and one group eating a traditional low-fat diet. None of the participants were restricted in calories and none had cardiovascular disease at the outset. Over the six years of the study, which was published in the New England Journal of Medicine in April 2013, the subjects in the two Mediterranean diet groups experienced 30 percent fewer major cardiovascular events, such as heart attacks, than those in the low-fat diet group.

How could the Mediterranean diet make such a difference so quickly? The short answer is that it provided excellent nutrition in all the areas the human body needs, which allowed the subjects' cells to function better and, therefore, age less. The diet also did not include the kinds of dietary indulgences, such as saturated fats and refined sugars, that make cells perform poorly or overtax them.

Scientists are learning more all the time about how your diet affects your health based on what different foods do to your cells. To make small changes that will have the biggest impact on your health, you need to know where to start, which means you need to know how bad food choices harm you and good food choices help you. Once you do, you can try to replace one or two not-so-healthy elements of your diet with something that will allow your cells to age more slowly.

In the following chapter, you'll find a rundown of the foods that cause the biggest problems in the typical American diet, with an explanation of how those foods age you, followed by descriptions of foods that will reduce oxidative stress, protect your telomeres, help suppress cancer genes, and so on. Use this information to become more mindful about what you decide to eat so you can make better choices that will make you feel and look younger, no matter what your age.

Cornering the Culprits

Scientific studies have identified a host of health conditions associated with Americans' eating patterns, but plenty of disagreement exists about what foods, in particular, are to blame. One reason is that it's hard to engineer a perfect food study in humans. Studies trying to assess the effect of one particular food, for example, can't rule out interactions with or effects of other food the test subject has eaten, and it's extremely difficult to construct a study in which every bit of food a person eats is controlled. When researchers ask people to fill out questionnaires about what they've eaten, meanwhile, there's always the possibility the subject doesn't remember everything he or she consumed.

Additionally, it's hard to weed out other influencing factors that might change a researcher's results. Studies that link sugary sodas to health problems later in life, for example, might be detecting issues that arise from obesity because people who drink a lot of sugary drinks tend to be overweight. Studies that blame highly refined, processed foods could be picking up on the absence of fruits and vegetables because often people who eat a highly processed diet do not fill their carts with produce. And studies that tie high cholesterol, inflammation, and other heart-unhealthy conditions to red meat could be detecting the effect of other harmful compounds that result from cooking food at high temperatures. Good researchers try to adjust their results to minimize the impact of other factors, but these issues remain a problem for scientists trying to conduct accurate human studies.

Nevertheless, a growing body of evidence points to several different kinds of food, as well as the amounts of those foods we consume, as contributing to ill health and premature aging. Many people know these foods aren't good for them, but that's not enough: if you really understand what they're doing to your body, you'll feel more motivated to start cutting back on them, a little bit at a time.

Scary Sugars

Who doesn't love an ice-cold lemonade or a perfect creamy cupcake? But these kinds of sweets seem to have moved from the realm of the occasional treat to the world of everyday indulgence. Sugary drinks, in particular, are piling the pounds on many Americans. Numerous studies have linked consumption of sugar-sweetened beverages to being overweight and a higher incidence of type 2 diabetes. For example, a study published in 2011 in *Hypertension* linked sugary drinks to high blood pressure, and a study published in the journal *Circulation* in March 2012 found the risk of coronary heart disease is increased by drinking sweetened beverages.

The good news is, Americans are actually consuming less sugar than they used to, largely because the consumption of sugary drinks and sodas has been declining in the past decade. But Americans still eat an average of 76.7 grams per day of so-called "added sugars." These are sugars that are added to foods to make them taste good, as a preservative, or to replace fat. Today's consumers don't like products with high fat content, so making them sweeter is one way to make them less fatty but still palatable. The result is the typical American diet includes almost 20 teaspoons added sugar a day (or a whole lot more if you drink a large Coke every day), and that doesn't include any sugar you may put in your coffee or sprinkle on your cereal.

Added sugars are empty calories—they have no nutritional value. Yet Americans get close to 15 percent of all their calories every day from these added sugars—that's twice what's recommended. And some people get much more than that.

> "The typical American diet includes almost 20 teaspoons added sugar a day."

The more calories you get from added sugars, the more likely it is you'll consume too many calories overall because you still need to eat enough food to provide all the nutrients you need. That makes it far more likely you'll gain weight. Here's an example: if you eat a piece of birthday cake at an afternoon office party, will you eat less at dinner because of it? Probably not. Rather, these kinds of "treat" calories pile on top of whatever else we're going to eat like whipped cream on a sundae.

Clock-Cheater Tip

If you should be eating 2,000 calories a day, you need to consume almost all of those calories in real food just to get the nutrients you need to stay healthy and keep your cells from aging. If you eat extra sugar, you use up some of your 2,000-calorie budget, leaving fewer calories to "spend" on nutrition. Then, to get all the vitamins and minerals you need, you'll have to eat more than your allotted 2,000 calories. To pay for those calories, you basically go into debt: you go over budget, gain weight, and become less healthy. You've borrowed from your future health.

And the science of sugar is also complicated, because sugar isn't just sugar. It comes in numerous chemical forms, including glucose, fructose, sucrose (table sugar), lactose, and maltose. Scientists are learning a lot about how the different molecular structures of these forms of sugar behave differently in the body.

The most common sugar added to processed foods is fructose, usually in the form of high-fructose corn syrup, which may be especially bad for you. Kimber Stanhope, nutritional biologist at the University of California, Davis, is one of many scientists targeting sugar with science. She has found several uniquely bad qualities about fructose. For example, Stanhope has found that fructose is more likely than the simple sugar glucose to be stored in the body as fat, especially as fat that settles around the midsection. Belly fat has been linked to chronic diseases such as type 2 diabetes and other conditions. Regular glucose does not settle around the midsection as fat.

The chemical structure in glucose, meanwhile, stimulates the production of leptin, a hormone produced by your fat cells that tells your brain when you're full so you know when to stop eating. Fructose, however, does *not* stimulate leptin. So you can keep eating or drinking a fructose-sweetened food or drink (like a soda or processed junk food), and your brain just won't get the same signal that you've had enough.

So you just plowed through a pack of Oreos? It's not lack of willpower—it's hormonal! That might make you feel better, but either way, the effect is the same: you've just eaten too many calories.

Processed foods, sugary drinks, sodas, and other foods that contain high-fructose corn syrup—and there are a lot of them—are contributing to America's weight and health problems in part because of the chemical structure of the sugar and the way it reacts in your body at the cellular level.

The source of the sugar you eat makes a big difference. Fructose may be the main sugar abundant in processed foods, but it's also the sugar found in fruit. Yet this kind of fructose isn't bad for you, because when you eat fructose in an apple or a plum, you are not only getting all the nutrients from that piece of fruit, you are getting fiber as well. And besides slowing your digestion so you absorb the sugar more slowly, guess what else fiber does? It stimulates the production of leptin—the hormone that tells your brain when you're full so you should stop eating.

> "So you just plowed through a pack of Oreos? It's not lack of willpower—it's hormonal!"

Think about how much of a difference fiber can make in how much you consume. To get the same number of calories as that large Coke from McDonald's, you'd have to eat about $3^1/_2$ apples—but you wouldn't do that because all the fiber in those apples would make you feel too full.

The "Bad" Carbohydrates

You want some carbohydrates in your diet; you just don't want too many of the wrong kinds. But that's exactly what Americans love to eat: anything made with refined, processed, white flour, such as cakes, cookies, breads, crackers, pizza crust, pasta, and tortillas, as well as white rice, potato chips, and many other snacks and processed foods.

But many studies have implicated refined carbs as a health hazard in the American diet, linking them to obesity and type 2 diabetes. A study published in 2011 in *The American Journal of Clinical Nutrition* also found that consumption of refined carbohydrates can lead to heart disease.

What's so bad about them? The grains used in these foods have been stripped of the parts that, in the original plant, contained all or most of the vitamins, minerals, and fiber. What's left is virtually void of nutrition. So like added sugars, refined sugars provide nearly empty calories and, therefore, increase the chances of weight gain. (Remember, *empty* calories tend to become *extra* calories.) Some foods, such as breakfast cereals, have select vitamins and minerals added back in, but not usually enough to equal the whole-grain version of flour. And again, the lack of fiber makes eating these carbohydrates similar to eating pure sugar: nothing tells you to stop.

More problematic is that the lack of fiber in most refined carbohydrates means they're quickly and easily digested, creating an immediate spike in the level of sugar flowing

> "*Empty* calories tend to become *extra* calories."

into your blood. That forces your body to quickly produce enough insulin to help digest all that sugar from your food. But that's not what your body was designed to do; it was designed to get sugar from plant sources, which would contain fiber to slow down the absorption of that sugar—and more stable insulin production.

Clock-Cheater Tip

Fiber helps your body digest your food slower so you feel full and your blood sugar stays more stable. That stability minimizes stress on your cells and keeps them healthier. So if you must have a sweet treat, make the portion a little smaller and eat something with plenty of fiber at the same time, such as berries, popcorn, or almonds. This trick, done consistently over time, will help minimize the effects of aging at the cellular level.

When you feed refined carbohydrates to your cells, it's a lot like facing an impossibly difficult deadline at work. Imagine walking into the office and finding out a project you've been working on has to be finished in just 2 hours. You fly into a panic, and pull every possible shortcut to get it done. The final version isn't especially polished, and you are a nervous wreck. That's your body after eating refined carbohydrates.

On the other hand, if you get to work and found out that you have 2 days to complete your project, you may still have a lot of work to do, but you would have enough time to make a plan, delegate tasks, and get it right. Not only would the final version be much cleaner, but you'd feel better about it and less stressed. That's how your body reacts when you eat whole grains.

The speed with which sugar from a food shows up in the bloodstream after eating is a measurement called glycemic index (GI), and the higher the GI, the more quickly the sugar from that food is absorbed. Consumption of high-glycemic foods—as most refined carbohydrates are—has been linked to higher rates of obesity, diabetes, and cardio-vascular disease, among other conditions, in numerous studies.

Bad things happen when your blood sugar levels are constantly rising and falling sharply: it can stimulate the creation of fat molecules, encourage inflammation (a risk factor for heart disease), and cause the body to become less sensitive to insulin. Because your body wasn't designed to handle yo-yoing levels of blood sugar, your cells don't handle it well. After a while, they become fatigued and don't respond as well to the presence of insulin. This insulin resistance keeps more glucose circulating in the blood than there should be and is considered a precursor to diabetes.

A diet full of processed, refined carbohydrates (picture a pastry for breakfast, pretzels for a snack, fast food for lunch, ice cream for a treat, and pizza for dinner) makes your cells age prematurely. It's what would happen to you if you walked into work every day and had a project due at noon. Pretty soon you'd feel exhausted, overwhelmed, and ready to quit.

> "A diet full of processed, refined carbohydrates ... makes your cells age prematurely."

Meaty Issues

The potentially harmful effects of red meat have been a big topic of debate. Some studies show red meat raises the risk of diabetes, heart disease, and various kinds of cancer, but other studies don't show these results.

The conflicting data in some scientific investigations of red meat highlight the limitations of food-specific studies and the degree to which they can be biased or misinterpreted. For one thing, people who eat a lot of red meat often have other unhealthy habits, such as not eating enough fruits and vegetables or not exercising regularly. And Americans consume so many different kinds of "red meat"—some fatty, some lean, some processed, some plain, some charred, some rare, and so on—it's difficult to pinpoint the cause and effect of any observed negative health consequences.

But compelling research suggests eating more than a small quantity of red meat—especially the processed variety—is harmful.

A large study from researchers at Harvard, published in 2012 in the journal *Archives of Internal Medicine,* analyzed data from two major studies of health professionals whose dietary and health habits had been tracked over 20 to 30 years. It was the first big-scale study done over a long period of time to assess the impact on premature death from consumption of red meat. The study found that just one moderate serving of red meat—about the size of a deck of cards—eaten every day was linked to a 13 percent increased risk of death from any cause. Consuming a daily portion of processed red meat (such as one hot dog or two slices of bacon) was associated with a 20 percent greater risk of death. The study also showed that the more red meat someone consumed, the greater their risk of death.

Another way to look at this data is to calculate how many people were affected. By that measure, the researchers estimate, nearly 1,000 of the approximately 24,000 people who died during the years studied would *not* have died if they had limited their red meat consumption to just half a serving a day or less. None of the subjects who died had any evidence of heart disease or cancer at the outset.

What is it in red meat that causes this effect? That's still unsettled. It's possible that red meat triggers multiple ill effects, but it also may behave differently in different people. The areas scientists are focusing on as the most likely culprits include the following:

High levels of saturated fat in red meat. Saturated fat has been linked to increased levels of LDL or "bad" cholesterol in the blood, a known risk factor for clogged arteries, heart attacks, and stroke.

Cancer-causing compounds in meats created when they're cooked at high temperatures, such as when they're fried and grilled. These compounds are formed when meat is exposed to open flames or when enzymes and sugars react with creatine (an enzyme derivative found in muscle) under high heat. These compounds have been linked to cancer in lab animals and also in some human studies.

Meat contains a type of sugar molecule not found in humans that prompts a reaction from the human immune system, possibly contributing to a state of chronic inflammation. Inflammation is widely attributed to conditions of aging, including heart disease, diabetes, and neuro-degenerative diseases such as Alzheimer's, and has been linked to regular consumption of red meat.

Many scientists who focus their research on aging and age-related conditions strongly suggest limiting consumption of red meat, especially processed red meat, as one way to minimize aging at the cellular level.

Excess Calories

Many Americans overeat and as a result, they carry around excess fat. Why is that so bad? What's wrong with a few extra pounds—or 20 or 30? Quite a lot, it turns out. Indeed, some of the nation's top aging experts say the biggest problem facing this country in terms of aging isn't *what* we eat as much as it is *how much* we eat.

"Lifespan projections are going down for the first time in recorded history in the United States," says Brian Kennedy, chief executive of the Buck Institute for Research on Aging outside San Francisco. "Our bodies just aren't evolved to deal with overnutrition. Our bodies are evolved to deal with undernutrition."

When we experience overnutrition, and the resulting buildup of fat cells—billions of them—we do not fare very well. Overweight and obese people tend to have higher rates of disease and die younger. But why?

Scientists once thought fat was just a storage mechanism for excess energy; if you ate too many calories, they ended up stored in fatty tissue to be used later if needed. But it turns out that fat cells are far more active than anyone had thought, secreting a variety of hormones that can have harmful effects around the body, ultimately leading to inflammation, heart disease, diabetes, and cancer.

> "'Our bodies just aren't evolved to deal with overnutrition. Our bodies are evolved to deal with undernutrition.'"

Eating too much also puts stress on your cells through increased oxidation. Remember that the mitochondria in your cells turn the food you eat into energy, in the process creating free radicals that can damage cells. Well, when you overeat, your mitochondria go into overdrive trying to process all that nutrition, creating an overflow of free radicals and oxidative damage within your cells. That, in turn, means the body's natural antioxidant enzymes have to work feverishly to rid the body of all those rogue radicals, explains Tom Slaga, professor of pharmacology at the University of Texas Health Science Center at San Antonio.

Not only is it difficult for those antioxidant enzymes to keep up, but many of those enzymes also perform other important jobs in your body, often in concert with other enzymes, proteins, or hormones. If they're getting overwhelmed just trying to clean up an overload of free radicals, they're unable to perform their other duties, which in turn can throw off other hormonal and enzyme balances in the body, creating a cascade of poor performance, damage, and aging. Imagine trying to keep your house clean with 10 slovenly occupants living in it. You'd spend all your time just tidying up their daily messes, and you'd never get around to dusting the shelves or washing the kitchen floor. That's what overeating does to your cells.

"By taking in too many calories, your whole metabolic system gets out of kilter," Slaga says.

> "Imagine trying to keep your house clean with 10 slovenly occupants living in it. You'd spend all your time just tidying up their daily messes .... That's what overeating does to your cells."

Aiming for the AGEs

A compelling new area of scientific study is the process of glycation when food is cooked. You may never have heard of glycation, but you see it every day: it's the chemical process that makes the crust form on a loaf of bread when it bakes in the oven, or that makes roasted meat turn deliciously brown, or that turns sugar to caramel. It makes food smell good and taste delicious, and although that might seem like a harmless—and yummy!—result of cooking, it has a serious downside.

What's actually happening during this browning process is protein and fat molecules are combining with sugar molecules to form complex chemical substances called advanced glycation end-products, or AGEs for short. These compounds are toxic to your cells.

"When [AGEs] get to your cells they create huge amounts of oxidative stress," said Dr. Luigi Ferrucci of the National Institute on Aging. "So it may be that the *way* we cook our food is also important."

Scientists have known about AGEs for a long time because they are found naturally in the bloodstream, created by glucose in the blood that has bound to fats or proteins, and accumulate in the body with age. But until recently, they were thought to be a problem primarily created when blood sugar levels got out of control, such as from diabetes. The presence of too much sugar in the blood means more sugar molecules are available to bind with proteins, aided by heat inside the body. The effect of increased AGEs in the body is one reason diabetes is so harmful to long-term health, leading to premature aging and age-related complications.

But now scientists have found that AGEs are present in much of what we eat. A series of studies performed by Dr. Helen Vlassara, director of the diabetes and aging division at Mount Sinai School of Medicine in New York City, found that high levels of AGEs detected in the bloodstream could actually be attributed to the consumption of AGEs in food.

Food prepared with very hot or drying heat stimulates the creation of these toxic compounds. Dr. Vlassara has found that when consumed, AGEs enter your cells, cause rampant production of free radicals, and exhaust your body's natural antioxidant defenses. That leaves your cells ill equipped to fight other causes of oxidative stress (much the way those antioxidant defenses are overwhelmed by eating too much food). The runaway oxidative stress caused by AGEs puts your immune system on a constant state of alert, causing chronic inflammation, which has been linked to heart disease, diabetes, and cancer.

> "The runaway oxidative stress caused by AGEs puts your immune system on a constant state of alert, causing chronic inflammation, which has been linked to heart disease, diabetes, and cancer."

Vlassara has spent 35 years studying AGEs, and only recently has the mainstream scientific community sat up and noticed, thanks to a string of remarkable animal and human studies she's published showing the harmful effects of consuming high levels of AGEs.

"We demonstrated that AGEs come largely from food, and if you cut them down, you prevent diabetes, kidney disease, vascular disease, wound healing gets better, the survival is longer," she explains.

And that's not all. AGEs aren't just pro-oxidants; they are also sticky and can bind to proteins such as cholesterol, making it stick to your arteries. They also cause collagen proteins to stick together, making them stiff and inflexible, leading to cataracts, stiff joints, and wrinkles. Vlassara and others have also linked the presence of high levels of AGEs to dementia, stroke, skin aging, and more.

What makes this problem especially serious now, Vlassara says, is that far more food today contains AGEs than just a few decades ago, when people ate more fresh, home-prepared meals. Today, many of the meals we eat in restaurants contain high levels of AGEs due to extreme heat used in cooking, along with butter and some fats that contain high levels of AGEs. Processed foods have high quantities of undetectable AGEs because high heat and drying techniques are often used in the manufacturing process.

"It's not really any of the particular components of the food that is the problem. It's the way they have been processed and modified so they are not in their natural state," Vlassara says. Because AGEs have so much intense flavor, and a kind of flavor people like, manufacturers have been increasingly adding synthetic AGEs to foods to make them taste good. "You see them as 'artificial flavors'" on ingredient lists, she says.

The presence of AGEs is measured with a scale called kilo units, or thousand units, per serving of food. Dr. Vlassara explains that the ideal daily consumption of AGEs is between 8,000 and 10,000 kilo units, but many people eat 15,000 to 25,000 kilo units, or more if they eat a lot of processed and fried foods. The result of that excess consumption of AGEs is a higher level of oxidative stress and inflammation at the cellular level, both of which lead to premature aging and disease.

Clock-Cheater Tip

Try reducing the AGEs in your food by using lower-temperature cooking methods, such as baking, steaming, stewing, and poaching. Using lemon- and vinegar-based marinades on meat before cooking also reduces aging, as does prebaking meat before grilling so it doesn't have to spend as much time over hot charcoal. Get more information at theage-lessway.com.

Vlassara has developed a program to reduce AGEs, which she says will help people achieve far better health profiles, even without reducing their caloric intake. The trick, she says, is to cook foods at lower temperatures and using gentler, slower cooking methods. For example, she says, a fried egg contains 1,240 AGE kilo units, while a scrambled egg, cooked at lower heat, contains only 75. Meanwhile, 3 ounces grilled chicken contains 5,500 AGE kilo units, while 3 ounces poached chicken has only 2,200.

The following table lists the AGE content of selected foods, in kilo units, with lower-AGE alternatives.

Food	AGEs
2 strips fried bacon	11,000
Vegetarian sausage link, 1 ounce	240
Broiled steak, 3 ounces	6,600
Pot roast, 3 ounces	1,605
American cheese, 1 ounce	6,600
Cheddar cheese, 1 ounce	1,605
Butter, 1 tablespoon	1,890
Mayonnaise, 1 tablespoon	1,400
Olive oil, 1 tablespoon	450
Chocolate peanut butter cup, 1 ounce	1,030
Chocolate-covered raisins	60
Potato chips, 1 ounce	865
Popcorn, microwave, no oil, 1 ounce	10
Rice Krispies, 1 ounce	600
Corn Flakes, 1 ounce	70

Source: The AGE-Less Way

Dr. Vlassara has compiled her research, along with low-AGE recipes, in a book called *The AGE-Less Way*. Perhaps the most interesting part of the book, however, is stories of several test subjects who dramatically improved their health by going on a low-AGE diet, consisting simply of different cooking methods, but not fewer calories. Vlassara believes many of the ailments we now treat with drugs can be treated with a change in food preparation. Indeed, the way our food is prepared and processed, she argues, is what has changed most dramatically in the American diet over the past 50 years, exactly coinciding with the alarming increase in many of the chronic diseases now plaguing the country, such as diabetes and heart disease.

"This theory is very new," she says, adding that it's been difficult to get other members of the scientific community, as well as funding sources, to buy into her research. But interest is rising in the field here and overseas, and more studies are showing promising results in a variety of areas.

Anyone with chronic back pain, for example, will be interested in a study published in May 2013, in which Vlassara and a team of researchers linked spinal disc degeneration in mice to the accumulation of AGEs in the spine. Treating the mice with drugs to minimize inflammation and the accumulation of AGEs either prevented or reduced spinal and disc degeneration in the mice. The study, the authors said, "may have broad public health implications."

Undoubtedly, you have not heard the last of AGEs.

Information Trumps Temptation

The previous sections seem to suggest that many of the foods Americans love—such as sweetened drinks (added sugars), cupcakes (made with white flour), grilled steaks (cancer-causing compounds), the all-you-can-eat bar (too many calories), and fried chicken (full of toxic AGEs)—should be off limits.

You don't need to totally wipe the slate clean of these foods to age well; you just need to start thinking more about which ones you really want and which ones you could sub out for something better, at least some of the time. The trick is to start with just a few small changes that aren't difficult to make, or even noticeable, and build them up over time.

For example, to reduce AGEs in your diet, you may not have to reduce the number of calories you consume. It may be enough to eat the same amount of food but prepared a different way, using lower heat. That's an easy and painless change.

If you must have a piece of chocolate or a cookie, eat some berries with it so the fiber in the berries can keep your blood sugar more stable and give your body a boost of antioxidants to help deal with the influx of sugar.

And the next time you find yourself choosing between fried chicken or baked chicken at a restaurant, stop and think about the AGEs in the fried chicken and what those compounds are doing to your cells. It will help you make the healthier decision.

Likewise, before you reach for a soda, picture the $3^1/_2$ apples you'd have to eat to equal the calories in that soft drink.

Eating to age well doesn't have to be about resisting temptation. Instead, use the information in this book to make better choices for your body— for your cells—by eating more of the foods that scientists know will help your cells age less.

"Eating to age well doesn't have to be about resisting temptation."

The next chapter lays out the science behind the best choices for your diet. The trick is to remember that you don't need to make these changes all at once, as you'll see from Jim's experience. He transformed his diet ever so slowly, and in the process, he transformed himself.

Antiaging Eating

Remember the studies on the Mediterranean Diet that were so beneficial to the subjects? The diet worked because the food they ate allowed all the mechanisms inside their cells to operate at an optimal level. Over time, eating like this adds up to feeling better, looking better, and aging less. So when you want to make a healthier choice—starting with once a day or even once a week—pick a food that will do some good at the cellular level and, therefore, help you age less and live more.

Eating to age well should be enjoyable. No one wants to go through life not enjoying or appreciating their food (that's why it's such a chore to go on a diet!). But it is possible to get more antiaging foods into your diet pretty easily, and even like it!

In this chapter, you learn what makes fruits and vegetables matter so much, how different sources of protein pack a punch, and how little things, like which oil you use to cook with, make a big difference. When you're eating to cheat the clock, there's no broken diet or bad decision. The goal is choosing foods that will make a difference in the long term. So if you don't eat the right foods at lunch, or at any time today, you can make a better choice at your next meal, or tomorrow. It takes time to change, and that's okay. If you make bad decisions for a day, or even a week, don't give up—it won't make a difference to how well you'll age. What does make a difference is adding up positive changes over time.

The Building Blocks

To be more mindful of your choices, you need to know what you're looking for, and why. Eating the right foods can keep your cells, your organs, your muscles, your skin, your brain, and your energy level youthful for years to come. So to start, here are the basic building blocks your body needs to maintain its performance and ability:

- Vitamins
- Minerals
- Protein
- Fiber
- Healthy fats
- Phytochemicals

Vitamins are natural chemical compounds used in small amounts in your body to perform specific, essential jobs. Vitamins interact with proteins and enzymes to govern your most basic cellular functions, including generating energy, developing and replicating correctly, and fighting infections and abnormal growth (cancer).

Minerals come from nonliving sources, such as rocks and metals. Plants absorb minerals from the soil, and the animals or people who eat the plants reap the benefits. Minerals are generally essential for more structural functions, including the formation of bones, teeth, cell membranes, the brain, blood cells, and hormones. Their roles are exceedingly widespread, complex, and not always well understood.

Protein is essential to life. When digested, it's broken down into its basic structure of amino acids, which then perform thousands of critical functions in your body. Your body makes some amino acids on its own, but it must obtain many required amino acids from plant- or animal-based protein-rich foods.

Fiber is the part of plants, legumes, or nuts that your body cannot digest, but even so, it performs several important functions when consumed. Fiber comes in two forms:

- Insoluble fiber
- Soluble fiber

Insoluble fiber, found in many vegetables, nuts, and whole grains, does not dissolve in water and moves through your body largely intact, gathering up the by-products of digestion and creating a constant movement of stool through the colon.

Soluble fiber, found in oats, lentils, nuts, and fruits and vegetables, dissolves in water to become gel-like in your body. This gel slows down how quickly your stomach empties, so you feel fuller longer, and also slows the digestion of sugar, leading to better insulin regulation. This kind of fiber also interferes with the absorption of dietary cholesterol, so it can help lower your "bad" cholesterol.

Healthy fats and phytochemicals are less well understood, but the science is getting clearer that certain types of fats, such as omega-3 fatty acids, help your cells perform better in a variety of ways. Meanwhile, myriad chemical compounds found in fruits and vegetables also are emerging as critical parts of your diet. They help your body maintain peak physical and mental functions by acting as antioxidants and interacting with the body's own defenses to improve their function.

For long-term health and slower aging, the food choices you make should flow from these building blocks. Yes, you want to eat less of the bad stuff (or maybe less in general, which I get to later), but eating foods that are good for you can go a long way toward helping your body handle the damage caused by other poor habits. The best part is that the more healthy foods you eat, the better you feel, so the more you will end up wanting them. Eventually, you'll find you won't want to reach for greasy, sugary, empty calories nearly as much, if at all.

Micronutrient Magic

Everyone knows they need a certain amount of vitamins and minerals, but few people really understand what these nutrients do in the body or why they're so essential. People figure if they aren't sick, they're probably getting enough vitamins and minerals.

But learning the role micronutrients play at the microscopic level is eye-opening and highly motivating: it truly makes you want to get enough of them. Although vitamins and minerals have been studied for decades, and an enormous amount of information about them exists, scientists are still discovering new ways they're involved in keeping us healthy and, in particular, keeping us young.

One such researcher is Dr. Bruce Ames, professor of biochemistry and molecular biology at the University of California, Berkeley. He has spent much of his career trying to figure out why our bodies are able to put up with so much when we're young but when we get older, we start to fall apart. If we can stay healthy and vigorous throughout our youth, what changes? Why can't we stay that way?

13 Essential Vitamins

According to the U.S. Food and Drug Administration, 13 vitamins are essential for human health: vitamins A, C, D, E, K, and the B vitamins folate, thiamin, riboflavin, niacin, pantothenic acid, biotin, vitamin B_6, and vitamin B_{12}.

Dr. Ames' extensive research points to the possibility that many people—even those who seem to have adequate diets—are slightly, but chronically, deficient in a host of essential vitamins and minerals. They may be getting enough vitamin C to avoid scurvy and enough vitamin D to prevent rickets, but they are deficient enough that it's wreaking long-term havoc on their health and vitality.

When you get just slightly less of the essential micronutrients you need by not eating enough fruits, vegetables, and other plant-based foods, Ames says, "you pay a price for it in long-term health."

Government data suggests he might be right. The following table shows, according to the U.S. Department of Agriculture (USDA), how the typical American female, age 31 to 50, falls short in the consumption of these micronutrients.

Vitamin/ Mineral	Good Sources	Recommended Daily Intake	Actual Daily Intake*
Calcium	Dairy products, broccoli, leafy greens	1,000 milligrams	850 milligrams
Vitamin D	Sunlight, egg yolks, fish oil	15 micrograms	3.6 micrograms
Vitamin E	Oils, nuts, dark leafy greens	15 milligrams	7 milligrams
Vitamin A	Milk, eggs, orange or green veggies	700 micrograms	550 micrograms
Iron	Meat, fish, lentils, beans, soy products	18 milligrams	13 milligrams
Magnesium	Whole grains, nuts, leafy greens, bananas	320 milligrams	260 milligrams

This is the mean daily intake, so half of U.S. women in this age group consume more than this amount, and half consume less.

In the *Proceedings of the National Academy of Sciences,* Dr. Ames reviewed years of scientific studies assessing the diseases and illnesses that have been associated with chronic deficiencies in various vitamins and minerals. The conditions and diseases mentioned are almost all ones we commonly associate with aging, such as:

- **Calcium, vitamin B$_{12}$, and zinc:** Deficiency can result in breakage of chromosomes.

- **Magnesium:** Deficiency can cause colorectal and other cancers, hypertension, osteoporosis, diabetes, and metabolic syndrome.
- **Vitamin D:** Deficiency associated with colon, breast, pancreatic, and prostate cancer, and with cardiovascular disease.
- **Thiamin (vitamin B₁):** Deficiency linked to brain dysfunction and diabetes.

Ames offers his research on vitamin K as a good example of how slight vitamin deficiencies can add up to premature aging and age-related disease.

Vitamin K? Who worries about vitamin K? That's exactly Ames' point. Found primarily in green, leafy vegetables, vitamin K isn't one many people think about, but it has multiple tasks in the body, including a critical role in blood clotting, both during fetal development and throughout life. When Ames bred mice that couldn't process vitamin K for blood coagulation, they quickly died, illustrating how critical the vitamin is for some bodily functions. But vitamin K plays a secondary role in increasing bone density and in the prevention of arterial calcification—jobs that are critical to good health later in life.

Going Green

Vitamin K is found in chlorophyll, the chemical that gives plants a dark green color. In your diet, you can get vitamin K from dark greens like spinach or kale, but also from other green foods, including cabbage, broccoli, and even green tea.

Scientists have discovered a range of proteins in the body that bind to calcium in the bloodstream. But it turns out they must have vitamin K to do their jobs. If you don't have enough vitamin K circulating in your blood, these proteins can't assume the right molecular structure to pick up calcium. That means loose calcium molecules that should have been carried away by these specialized calcium-cleaners are instead left circulating in your body. Some of this excess calcium ends up sticking to the walls of your arteries. This buildup of calcium in your vascular system can play a significant role in the development of atherosclerosis, or hardening of the arteries, one of the most common health problems in aging.

"How do you prevent the calcification of your arteries? From vitamin K. Where does this vitamin K come from? Fruits and vegetables," says Dr. Maret Traber, nutritional biochemist at the Linus Pauling Institute, the micronutrient research center at Oregon State University.

How big a deal is this? Possibly huge. According to government data, men in particular are chronically, moderately deficient in vitamin K. Between the ages of 30 and 50, men get an average of about 106 micrograms a day of vitamin K, according to the USDA, but 120 micrograms is considered adequate. This slight deficit won't cause problems today, but over the long term, scientists believe, it is contributing to cardiovascular disease, the number-one cause of death in the United States.

For every vitamin K story like this, there are dozens of others related to other specific vitamins and minerals. For example, Dr. Ames is on a crusade to get people to eat enough magnesium, which it turns out is critical to more than 300 metabolic processes in your body, including energy production and enzyme creation. Magnesium is found primarily in whole grains, nuts, and green leafy vegetables. The typical American adult gets about 80 percent of the recommended amount of magnesium a day.

"ATP [the chemical energy used by cells] has magnesium in it; all the DNA repair enzymes have magnesium in them," Ames said. "But the whole country is starving for magnesium."

To slow the aging process, it's important to get enough of all the recommended vitamins and minerals—even the ones you haven't heard of. To find out how much you should be getting, look at the government's Dietary Reference Intakes, which are based on decades of scientific testing. Log on to the USDA's Food and Nutrition Information Center website at fnic.nal.usda.gov/dietary-guidance to learn more.

Mandatory Minerals

According to the FDA, your body requires these minerals: calcium, chromium*, copper*, iodine*, iron*, magnesium, manganese*, molybdenum*, phosphorus, potassium, selenium*, sodium (chloride), and zinc.* (*Needed only in trace quantities.)

The best way to boost your intake of vitamins and minerals is to eat more fruits and vegetables. That simple act alone slows the aging process. Taking a multivitamin can also be helpful, of course, but plant-based foods do so much more than any pill ever could. The vitamins and minerals found in food come in exactly the right chemical form your body can use, which is not true of many supplement versions. As the foundation of human diets for millennia, fruits and vegetables are uniquely powerful in your body and provide the best support for your cells to stay healthy and age less.

In fact, when looking at the different nutrient building blocks your body needs, it's pretty obvious that plant-based foods give you the biggest bang for your buck. A varied diet of fruits, vegetables, grains, legumes, and nuts can provide all the vitamins, minerals, fiber, phytochemicals, fats, and protein your body needs. Nothing else you eat can do that.

"A varied diet of fruits, vegetables, grains, legumes, and nuts can provide all the vitamins, minerals, fiber, phytochemicals, fats, and protein your body needs. Nothing else you eat can do that."

That doesn't mean you should become a vegetarian. But it does mean that when fruits and vegetables play a major role in your diet, you will be healthier and probably live longer. Many studies have shown marked improvement in the health and mortality in numerous measurable ways in people who have boosted the amount of fruits and vegetables consumed.

Of course, the opposite is also true. If you do *not* eat enough fruits and vegetables, you're doing more long-term damage than you may think: just as Dr. Ames says, you're slowly robbing your body of the natural chemical and molecular compounds it must have to remain healthy and strong as you age.

Phytochemical Phenoms

It's not just the fiber, vitamins, and minerals that make fruits and vegetables so powerful, though. The huge number of less-well-known *phytochemicals* (*phyto* comes from the Greek word for "plant") also have important and beneficial physiological effects. Known more commonly as antioxidants, these chemicals, although not as well understood as vitamins and minerals, are also emerging as critical for their healthful effects.

A few years ago, only the super-committed health nuts among us knew about antioxidants. Now they're everywhere. Drink pomegranate juice! Eat blueberries! Antioxidants have become the latest healthy food buzzword among marketers, who have succeeded in letting many people know that antioxidants are something they should consume freely and often.

But many of the same people who are buying antioxidant-laden food still don't know what an antioxidant actually is, or what one does. You might know they fight free radicals. But do you know what a free radical is? Could you explain it to, say, your mother? So here you go: a free radical is a molecule—often an oxygen molecule—that's lost one electron, which makes it unstable and causes it to bounce around inside a cell and damage its internal structures. An antioxidant is a compound or molecule that binds to a free radical, making it stable again.

Scientists haven't yet finished unraveling the secrets of these magic molecules, and they may never fully understand the complexities involved. But they are learning more every day about how these powerful compounds act as nature's cell purifiers, ridding them of pollution, repairing damage, and generally keeping them in tip-top shape. You can't see or feel the effects of antioxidants when they're actually working, but they add up. Over time, cells that have been nourished with high doses of antioxidants are healthier and younger-looking. If your cells are healthier and younger-looking, it just makes sense that you will be, too.

> "These powerful compounds act as nature's cell purifiers, ridding them of pollution, repairing damage, and generally keeping them in tip-top shape."

Antioxidants have scientific names such as polyphenols, turpenoids, and carotenoids—some of which you may have seen written about or mentioned on food packaging. There are thousands of antioxidants, and more are being discovered all the time. Many of them contribute the color to fruits and vegetables, so they tend to be found in especially high concentrations in the skin of fruit such as apples and grapes.

Some of these phytochemicals have molecular structures that give them antioxidant properties—that is, they can lend an electron to a free radical so it will become stable and stop bouncing around inside a cell, causing damage (called oxidative stress). But recent research has uncovered what may be an even more critical role for the antioxidants you eat: they induce your body to make more of its own antioxidants that are naturally more effective at stopping oxidative stress than antioxidants you eat.

"This is particularly true for some carotenoids and flavonoids— they're not particularly good antioxidants in the traditional sense," says Tufts antioxidant researcher Blumberg. Rather, many of these phytochemicals stimulate production of a natural enzyme, like superoxide dismutase, which "quenches free radicals and does a better job of it, and it's generally right where you want it to be."

This process happens in a millisecond, but it's going on constantly, so the more you boost your antioxidant intake, the more free radical–fighting power your body has. The effect appears to be linear—that is, the more you consume, the more free radical–fighting compounds appear in your blood. One study in particular, performed at the

USDA Arkansas Children's Nutrition Center and published in the
Journal of the American College of Nutrition, measured the presence
of free radical–absorbing compounds in the human bloodstream.
Volunteers were asked to eat meals containing various fruits such
as cherries, prunes, kiwi, red grapes, strawberries, and blueberries
and then researchers measured the antioxidant levels in their blood.
The results showed that several different kinds of fruit caused big
spikes in the antioxidant capacity of the subjects' blood, including
blueberries, kiwi, and the tropical acai berry.

Clock-Cheater Tip

To boost your intake of antioxidants, wash your fruits
and vegetables thoroughly and eat the skin with the
flesh. The skin often has the highest concentration of
phytochemicals.

By contrast, in a separate part of the study, the volunteers were
also given a shake high in carbohydrates, protein, and fat, but no
antioxidants. After drinking the shake, all the volunteers showed a
measurable decline in the availability of antioxidants in their blood.

The study's conclusion was simple: eat at least some antioxidant-rich
foods with every meal.

But pinning down what or how much you should eat is incredibly
tricky. Scientists are increasingly realizing that the human body
responds best to a *combination* of different antioxidants, and there
are so many, it's impossible to tease out the relationships among
them. These different phytochemicals interact with each other and
with your body's own antioxidant systems in ways that aren't fully
understood. The science of antioxidants, some scientists say, is about
as developed today as it was for vitamins 100 years ago.

"There are thousands, maybe about 10,000, different phytochemicals,
at least that we know about so far, and which ones are the most
important ones? Well, I don't know," says Dr. Blumberg. "With 10,000
compounds, there's no way to have an adequate placebo and no time
or money to do a clinical study on each of these chemical compounds
for 30 or 40 years to have the hard outcome evidence."

Yet people want to know what to do and what to eat, so researchers are plugging away in labs, coming up with amazing results they can't always fully explain. In one study published in *The Journal of Neuroscience,* old rats fed a diet boosted with the extracts of several fruits and vegetables not only stopped, but even reversed, the signs and symptoms of aging in their brains. A similar result was found in research on dogs published in the journal *Neurobiology of Aging.*

Blumberg believes that as humans evolved over tens of thousands of years, largely eating plant-based food, they developed systems that capitalized on the defense mechanisms used in plants themselves. In their original plant sources, antioxidant compounds perform such functions as protecting plants from ultraviolet radiation, pests, and fungi.

"As we ate these foods we started taking advantage of the protective effects they had in plants, to be protective in us," Blumberg says. Lutein is a good example. This carotenoid antioxidant, found in egg yolks and also various fruits and vegetables, especially dark leafy greens such as kale and spinach, appears to help retard age-related macular degeneration, which causes progressive blindness in the elderly. In the eye, lutein filters out damaging blue wavelengths from light. "Well, guess what?" Blumberg says. "In the plant, it protects it from ultraviolet radiation."

The breadth of research on dietary antioxidant consumption (that is, from foods as opposed to supplements) in humans is growing dramatically, and so are the promising discoveries.

For example, Dr. Trygve O. Tollefsbol, molecular biologist at the University of Alabama, was blown away by experiments he did in lab animals using sulforaphane, a powerful antioxidant found in cruciferous vegetables such as broccoli and cabbage, as well as in soy and green tea. In a study on lab mice, published in 2011 in the journal *Clinical Epigenetics,* Dr. Tollefsbol found that a diet rich in sulforaphane showed epigenetic changes to their DNA structure that suppressed genes for cancer. How that translates to humans is unclear, but other research suggests the effects are playing out today in some populations. A 2006 study, published in the *Journal of the National Cancer Institute,* found that many Polish immigrants to the United States experienced far greater rates of breast cancer after just one generation of arriving here. The researchers concluded that the change was related to the decreased consumption of cabbage: Poles eat three times more cabbage than Americans.

Only in Okinawa

Compelling evidence of the beneficial effects of antioxidant consumption comes from a study of the island of Okinawa, Japan, where many men and women in their 70s, 80s, 90s, and older are physically fit, independent, strong, active, and disease free. A team of doctors from Okinawa International University found several identifiable behaviors that differ from the typical Western lifestyle—especially the fact that their diet is based largely on antioxidant-rich fruits, vegetables, and spices, along with seaweed, fish, and pork. The Okinawans' carbohydrate consumption comes not from rice, as in the typical Japanese diet, but almost entirely from the antioxidant- and vitamin-rich sweet potato. As a result of their diets, Okinawans have a much higher antioxidant capacity in their blood than Westerners do, and even higher than people in the rest of Japan.

Based on his research, Dr. Tollefsbol recommends people eat plenty of cruciferous vegetables, such as broccoli, cauliflower, and cabbage, and cook them as minimally as possible. He has found similar epigenetic benefits from green tea and suggests that people drink 2 or 3 cups a day. There's much more research to do, but the outlines of an "epigenetics diet" are starting to emerge, he says.

A Whole Lot of Help

In survey after survey, Americans say they want to eat more whole grains. In practice, though, only about 11 percent of the grains most Americans eat come from whole-grain sources. This is making them grow older, faster.

More and more research is proving how essential whole grains are in helping your body stave off the effects of aging. The fiber in whole grains slows your digestion and keeps blood sugar levels more stable. Antioxidants in whole grains fight the aging effects of oxidative stress. And whole grains contain many vitamins and minerals, which your cells must have if they are going to stay healthy for the long term.

Take a kernel of wheat as an example, which is used in its entirety in whole-wheat flour. The outer layer is called the bran, the seed is called the germ, and the endosperm is the rest of the plump interior. Where is most of the nutrition? In the bran and the seed—the parts that are discarded when making white flour. The bran contains fiber, minerals such as magnesium and selenium, as well as B vitamins. The germ, which is the embryo of a new wheat plant, has vitamins E, A, and K; more B vitamins; as well as protein, fiber, and healthy fats.

> "Where is most of the nutrition [in a kernel of wheat]? In the bran and the seed—the parts that are discarded when making white flour."

Studies have shown that boosting consumption of whole grains such as oats, popcorn, brown rice, rye, bulgur, and quinoa reduces the risk of heart disease and diabetes and cools inflammation, among other benefits that can lead to healthier aging. Whole grains can even affect the way your genes work, according to a Finnish study published in 2007 in *The American Journal of Clinical Nutrition*. In the study, overweight individuals with metabolic syndrome were fed a diet that included whole-grain rye. After 12 weeks, the researchers found decreased activity in 71 genes related to cell death and insulin resistance.

Adding more whole grains to your diet is getting easier because more such products are being sold in supermarkets. When you find ones you like, be sure you eat them instead of refined grains. A study published in 2010 in *The American Journal of Clinical Nutrition* found that increasing whole-grain consumption reduced the amount of fat around people's midsections, which is thought to be a trigger for cardiovascular disease and type 2 diabetes. The effect was negated, though, in people who ate more whole grains but didn't reduce their consumption of refined grains.

This simple substitution is an easy way to make your diet work for you and keep you healthier for years. It's not about sacrifice; it's about changing your habit. Take it a step at a time. If the last piece of whole-wheat bread you tried didn't appeal to you, try a different brand. Start with just one substitution a day—use whole-wheat bread instead of white bread or brown rice instead of white rice, for example—and when you get used to it, you can add another. Every little bit helps.

Proactive Protein

We've already looked at why reducing red meat in your diet can be a good way to reduce your risk of cardiovascular disease. But what should you eat instead? Many people eat a lot more protein than they need, and the trend has increased with the popularity of high-protein diets. According to the USDA, the typical man over age 30 needs 56 grams protein a day, and the typical woman that age needs 46 grams. There are lots of places to get that protein, and some are healthier than others.

Leaner choices such as chicken, fish, egg whites, beans, and fat-free dairy provide plenty of protein. They also often have other beneficial compounds linked to improving your health as you age.

A study recently published in the journal *Stroke* assessed the impact of dietary protein on the risk of stroke in a large population followed for 22 and 26 years. Not surprisingly, the study found that intake of red meat increased the risk of stroke. Then it looked at how that risk went down if just one serving of red meat a day was replaced with a different source of protein. It found that replacing one serving of red meat a day with poultry lowered the risk of stroke by 27 percent. Eating fish or nuts instead of red meat once a day lowered the risk by 17 percent.

"Replacing one serving of red meat a day with poultry lowered the risk of stroke by 27 percent."

What this study shows is that your protein choice is a great place to start making minor changes to your diet that can have a big impact. To get the most benefit from this part of your plate, try to mix it up so you get the nutritional benefits of each kind of protein. It's also a great way to figure out what you really like and can go on eating for years to come.

Poultry is a complete protein that provides all the different amino acids your cells need to create new proteins, and it's low in fat and calories. But how you eat it matters: chicken is often prepared in cream sauces or fried, both of which cancel out its great qualities. Instead, grab a rotisserie chicken at the supermarket (but throw out the skin!). Or poach a whole chicken with lots of onions, carrots, and celery; it makes wonderful chicken stock you can use for soup and healthy cooking, and the tender, poached meat is great in soups, salads, and sandwiches. (Plus it's very low in AGEs!) Or try the recipe for Quick Baked Lemon Chicken Breasts later in the book for another tasty, healthy option.

Seafood can be a great choice for complete protein that contains all the essential amino acids. But again, avoid deep-fried and pan-fried preparations to get the full benefits of the fish. Broiling and baking are great options. Oily fish such as salmon and mackerel also provide high levels of good fats such as omega-3 fatty acids.

Omega-3 Fatty Acids

Omega-3 fatty acids are used for many normal bodily functions, including blood clotting. As essential fatty acids, omega-3s must come from the diet, and sources include fatty fish, walnuts, vegetable oil, flax, and dark leafy greens. Omega-3s (with specific names DHA, ALA, and EPA) have been shown in studies to reduce the risk of death, heart attacks, and stroke. They also may reduce inflammation and the risk of cancer. Few of us get enough omega-3s. Aim for one serving of an omega-3 fatty acid–rich food every day, or take a fish oil supplement.

Beans and legumes contain large quantities of fiber, vitamins, and minerals along with big servings of protein. Plus they are complex carbohydrates that release their energy in your body slowly over time, keeping you fuller longer. They won't make your blood sugar levels gyrate, either. Adding beans into your diet is easy and inexpensive. At first, you can try eating a smaller portion of animal protein and supplementing with beans or lentils on the side. Or throw some chickpeas in your salad or pasta dish.

Because beans and legumes often lack at least one essential amino acid, if they're your only protein source, you want to eat them with whole grains that will provide that missing nutrition. Black beans and brown rice, hummus and whole-wheat pitas, or peanut butter on whole-wheat bread are great combinations that provide a complete— and delicious!—source of protein.

Other good sources of healthy protein include low-fat and nonfat dairy products, such as yogurt and skim milk, and nuts. Most people wouldn't eat nuts as a main source of protein, but they are a healthy choice if you don't eat too many. Small servings are okay, though, because nuts are nutrient dense, packing lots of protein and healthy fats in a small package. Instead of eating higher-fat sources of protein, sprinkle nuts on your cereal, put them in your pasta, toss them with salads, or add them to stir-fries.

> "Every small step you take in the direction of cell-boosting foods will add up to more time on the clock."

Remember that every small step you take in the direction of cell-boosting foods will add up to more time on the clock. You can do just a little bit here and there, and it can still mean real change.

Cutting Consumption

Remarkably, scientists have known for years how to slow down the aging process: eat less.

Actually, eat a lot less.

A dietary program called *caloric restriction*—eating at least 30 percent fewer calories than the typically recommended level—is the only mechanism that has been proven, scientifically, to slow aging. Caloric restriction has induced longer lifespans in mice and other lab animals, and the effect is relatively easy to re-create. Researchers still don't know all the ways caloric restriction works, but one theory is fairly simple: if metabolism damages cells through oxidative stress, then fewer calories consumed means fewer calories burned and less cell damage.

But that's not the whole story. Aging experts now know that low food levels also do something beneficial to the body's complex system of protective enzymes and hormones, kicking these systems—or pathways, as they're known—into high gear. When food is scarce, these systems go into overdrive ridding the body of toxins of all kinds, including environmental, chemical, and heavy metals that can damage cells over time. During periods of caloric restriction, the brain also generates new neurons, and existing brain tissue becomes more resistant to degeneration. And finally, enzymes are produced that protect DNA inside cells from damage.

Testing caloric restriction in humans over a long period of time isn't easy, and it's certainly not a great way to live—although some people do. Adherents of caloric restriction even have their own association. But some top aging experts don't think this diet is such a great idea.

"I actually think a lot of those people are probably malnourished," said Dr. Brian Kennedy, chief executive of the Buck Institute for Aging Research outside San Francisco and a widely published biologist who has extensively studied human aging. "When we feed [mice] in the lab, they get all the nutrients they need in their diet; we know how to put exactly what they need in their pellets. When people do it ... if they're eating 1,500 calories a day, it would be very hard to get everything you need in terms of nutrition."

But caloric restriction remains highly seductive for scientists because it gives them a way to study the factors that extend life and try to replicate them. A huge discovery was made in 2009, when a drug was discovered that mimics the effect of caloric restriction. In a coordinated experiment, three different labs tested a drug called Rapamycin on aging mice. It didn't seem especially promising at first; the study got started later than it was supposed to, so the mice colonies got old. When testing finally got underway, the mice were the equivalent of about 60 human years old and beginning to show signs of old age. It didn't seem like a great way to determine if a drug could retard aging.

But to everyone's surprise and delight, all three labs reported the same outcome—which is highly unusual in scientific research. Rapamycin induced the same cascade of cellular responses as caloric restriction, dramatically increasing the lifespan of the mice by 28 percent in males and 38 percent in females. This set of longevity-increasing reactions was named the TOR pathway, for Target of Rapamycin. That seminal experiment has opened up a new era of research into Rapamycin and its derivatives, as well as the TOR pathway and what makes it work.

> "All three labs reported the same outcome—which is highly unusual in scientific research. Rapamycin ... dramatically [increased] the lifespan of the mice."

But if you're hoping to run out and get yourself some Rapamycin, you'll have to wait. The drug has side effects in humans: for one, it suppresses the immune system. In fact, it's currently used as a drug in human organ transplant patients to prevent organ rejection. It's also used as a cancer drug. And even if scientists can figure out a way to make Rapamycin safe as an antiaging drug for humans, those who study the drug—and Dr. Kennedy is one of them—don't foresee such a simple medical solution to aging. More likely is that a range of drugs would work on certain aging mechanisms in certain people, but probably only in the context of a healthy diet and lifestyle, Kennedy predicts.

"I don't know if Rapamycin is the right answer, but what I do know is if you have ten of those drugs, one of them will be the right answer. So the field is emerging and you're going to see a whole list of drugs that have these benefits come down the pipe," Kennedy said. "I don't think it's going to replace encouraging them to exercise and eat right, but I think it'll augment healthspan—make people healthy longer."

Like many aging experts, Dr. Kennedy is fascinated by the effect of caloric restriction and has lately been especially interested in a different kind of energy restriction called *intermittent fasting*. This appears to have the same benefits as traditional caloric restriction but is easier for humans to achieve. Animal studies have been very promising, so now more scientists are testing the potential benefits in humans.

Effective Fasting

Have you ever had a day where you just got too busy to eat and perhaps went all day, or a large part of the day, without food? You didn't realize it at the time, but that period without eating—even if you felt fatigued or ravenous—was actually helping your cells.

Scientists have discovered that going with no food, or almost no food, for a day or two every so often, maybe once a week, has many of the same beneficial effects as consistently limiting the amount of food you eat. But with intermittent fasting, you eat normally on the days you're not fasting. It doesn't work if you make up the lost calories by gorging on the other days, or if you go too long without eating, or if your fasting days are too close together. And it doesn't work unless you eat just the barest minimum on fasting days, such as some vegetables and tea, perhaps, for a maximum of about 500 to 600 calories. This diet increases insulin sensitivity, decreases belly fat, raises the level of beneficial hormones in the blood, and more.

Clock-Cheater Tip

If you want to try intermittent fasting, you can always ease into it. Try skipping lunch once a week for a while, and go up to 2 days in a row. But don't overeat when you're not fasting. Just go back to eating normally. Over time, you may lose weight, but the research suggests the benefits could be profound in terms of long-term health.

Subjects in Manchester, England, who followed an intermittent fasting program for 6 months in which they ate 600 calories a day for 2 days and then ate normally for 5 days reported that after the first 2 weeks, the program was easy to stick with. Some subjects even stayed on it after the study period was over because they lost weight and it made them feel better.

"The psychology of it is if you know you can eat normally for five days, you can get through two days not eating much," said Dr. Mark Mattson, senior investigator for the National Institute on Aging, who runs its neuroscience lab. Mattson is one of the nation's leading researchers on Alzheimer's, a disease that afflicts his own father. He began studying caloric restriction because of the beneficial effects it seems to have on the brain.

In his current research, Mattson has found that "intermittent fasting may increase the number of mitochondria in nerve cells" in the brain. That would provide more energy to the brain and possibly increase cognitive ability. This could be one mechanism that makes animals on an intermittent fasting diet show improved learning and working memory. In the fall of 2013, Mattson will initiate a study testing various cognitive measures in people ages 55 to 70 after two months on an intermittent fasting diet, which is typically more than enough time to start seeing clear protective benefits in the brain, he said.

Intermittent fasting also appears to increase the production of chaperone proteins, which help keep proteins in the brain properly folded, an important characteristic in the prevention of brain-degenerating diseases. In addition, Mattson found that fasting stimulated the production of a protein called brain-derived neurotrophic factor, or BDNF, which promotes the growth and survival of neurons in the brain. The brain actually created new connections as a result of the stress from intermittent fasting.

"[BDNF] plays a critical role in learning and memory and particularly may play an important role in protecting synapses during aging, preserving their function and plasticity and therefore preserving learning and memory," Dr. Mattson says. BDNF declines during normal aging, and more so in Alzheimer's patients, he says, so anything that boosts production of this critical protein will help maintain brain health through the years.

> "Intermittent fasting ... enhanced the ability of nerve cells in the brain to cope with stress and resist disease."

Vigorous exercise also promotes the production of BDNF. So does intellectual stimulation. That's thought to be one of the reasons, Mattson said, why a moderate diet, regular exercise, and continual intellectual engagement are known to help prevent the onset of Alzheimer's.

Why intermittent fasting initiates these protective cellular and systemic responses isn't well understood. Mattson's theory is that it's an adaptation left over from an era when humans were hunters and gatherers and food was frequently scarce. During these periods, you had an increased chance of survival if you had the capacity to work harder for food, remember where good food sources were, and withstand the stress of going out and securing it. So the human species developed ways of enhancing performance when food caloric intake plummeted. He also said that fasting seems to work differently from caloric restriction—and possibly better in some ways—because the cells spend a period of time being stressed, which throws protective mechanisms into action, but then a longer period of time resting, recovering, and doing the normal work of living. "The intermittent aspect is important," Mattson says.

The effect of intermittent fasting is being increasingly well documented, and scientists are looking with new enthusiasm at this dietary pattern as a possible way to slow human aging, although they caution that more research is needed to fully understand the pros and cons.

"I think it's going to be possible to extend lifespan by doing that," says Dr. Kennedy of the Buck Institute. "You go on this special diet where you have bars and shakes for like three days every month, I think it's going to be very effective."

Intermittent fasting is also being studied as a possible way to make cancer treatment more effective. The protective proteins released throughout the body as a result of intermittent fasting appear to reduce DNA damage, so doctors think it might help limit the harm caused to regular cells by chemotherapy treatment, which extensively damages DNA, allowing for higher doses to be administered with fewer side effects.

How much fasting is enough? Numerous schedules have been tried and proposed: alternate days with just a few hundred calories, or 2 days a week, or 1 day a week. But the data is still too scarce to make a true recommendation. Dr. Mattson says even stretching out the time between meals—sort of a modified fast—could have beneficial effects. Let yourself get really hungry. Mattson himself skips breakfast, exercises at lunch instead of eating, then has whatever he wants for dinner. "I basically eat for three straight hours," he says, only half joking. Kennedy, of the Buck institute, eats largely the same way, skipping lunch entirely, although he has a small breakfast.

"Even stretching out the time between meals—sort of a modified fast—could have beneficial effects. Let yourself get really hungry."

This may be yet another way my husband is following the science and reaping the benefits. Jim regularly has days at work, especially if he's in a trial, that are so busy he can't eat lunch, or he might not eat until 4 in the afternoon, at which point he usually eats a very small lunch so he doesn't ruin dinner. And even on normal days, he never eats between meals—there's just no time. Mattson says this eating schedule may very well be producing a protective effect in his cells.

Overcoming Overeating

Letting yourself get hungry, much less fasting, is totally at odds with the way most Americans eat today. Yet many aging scientists and nutritionists argue that one of the biggest problems facing America when it comes to aging is simply that we eat too much. According to the Centers for Disease Control, if people continue to gain weight at the rate they are now, 42 percent of the population will be obese in the year 2030. Obese people do not age well. Typically they develop a host of health problems that can greatly affect their lifespans—and healthspans.

Clock-Cheater Tip

If you don't know how many calories you eat in a day, spend a few days adding them up. Do this even if you aren't on a diet or think you don't overeat! You can use any calorie-counter book or website. Knowing how much you eat is crucial to your health because it can easily creep up when you aren't paying attention (willfully or not!). Just knowing this information makes you more aware of the food decisions you make.

People overeat for many reasons, and knowing more about some of the forces at work can help you push back and start eating a healthier amount of food—or simply resist temptation to overeat whenever it happens. If you need to cut back your total food intake, you don't have to make a dramatic change all at once. You can do it gradually, which will not only make it easier to change, but also make your changes more likely to stick. However you approach it, being more aware of the amount of food you eat, when you eat it, and why can help reverse the trend.

Taming Cravings

If you consistently overeat—consuming more than 2,000 calories a day, for example, or maybe 1,700 if you're sedentary—you have probably tried cutting back before, perhaps unsuccessfully.

But there are ways you can reduce how much you eat that are less difficult if you take a more long-term approach. It begins with a better understanding of the science behind the human appetite, which begins in the brain. This knowledge is especially helpful when your appetite becomes a problem.

"Working with people with all sorts of addictions, food is the one that is the hardest," explains Dr. Kelly McGonigal, PhD research psychologist and lecturer at Stanford University. Dr. McGonigal studies the biological basis for people's motivations and looks for ways to route around those ingrained habits and psychological urges. She has written and lectured extensively about the mind-body connection, including her recent book, *The Willpower Instinct: How Self-Control Works, Why It Matters, and What You Can Do to Get More of It.*

The reason our desire for food can be so hard to control is because our brains are wired, from way back in evolutionary history, to compel us to consume excess stores of energy whenever possible. But sometimes those signals go into overdrive—or "crazed consumption mode," as McGonigal calls it. When that happens, these signals can dominate everything else we feel or notice: it becomes all about the food.

But these deeply ingrained prehistoric signals don't have to control what we do. They're just pathways in the brain (albeit strong ones), and they can be changed. Dr. McGonigal says that with a little self-awareness and effort, you can begin to short-circuit those unwanted messages, literally confusing them and eventually wearing them down, sort of like overwriting data on a computer or DVD.

The first step is recognizing that the way you feel about food, especially if you crave it or obsess about it, is not a symptom of weakness, but a sign of brain signals run amok. To effectively deal with this challenging, all-consuming situation, you can't just overcome your desire to eat whatever it is; you have to change the signals in your brain.

As part of this process, it helps to recognize that "the act of consuming does not turn off the desire to consume," McGonigal says. For example, let's say you ate a cupcake at a party, and it was delicious. But now you want a second one from the huge platter of cupcakes just brought out. You can't stop thinking about, and wanting, another cupcake, even when you're talking to people at the party.

One of the trickiest parts of these disruptive messages from your brain is that they feel like they'll go away if you eat that cupcake. You believe you'll feel satisfied and be able to move on. But the opposite is usually true. The act of eating that second treat simply reinforces the signal telling you to eat. By eating the second cupcake, you've let your brain know that excess energy stores (calories) are available, and because your brain *wants* you to overconsume, you're right back where you started. You are Charlie Brown, and Lucy is controlling your cravings. Every time you try to kick it, she pulls it away.

One way to try to rewire this inner signal is to "put some distance between you and ... the temptation" by physically moving away from it, says McGonigal. "The brain starts to get the message that you are not approaching ... that you are saying no." This purposeful act won't eliminate the craving, but it will begin to dull the brain's frenzy to consume, as it simultaneously processes the fact that the food is going away.

You can also try "surfing the urge," as it's called: focus your attention as much as you can on your desire for that cupcake, really paying attention to what it feels like inside your body to be consumed by the desire to eat it. That inner-awareness process also works sort of like crossing wires in your brain.

"Turning your attention and awareness to the experience of wanting it screws up what's happening in the brain," McGonigal says. "It transforms the brain's ability to create this uncontrollable urge to consume."

These kinds of brain-signal awareness techniques take some practice, but scientists have found that the more you notice them, and really pay attention to how they feel, the more control you will have over them. "Accept that inner experiences are not things that you choose," says McGonigal.

This is one of McGonigal's key insights about willpower, which I discuss more extensively later in the book.

Snack Attack

We have become a nation of snackers, and it's certainly not doing anyone any good. According to the USDA, Americans eat an average of 2.2 snacks a day, and in the past 30 years, the number of people who snack rose from 59 percent to 90 percent, encouraged, perhaps, by the now commonly offered warning that it's not good for you to let your blood sugar get too low because it decreases cognitive performance and saps physical energy. Another recent book, *Willpower* by Roy F. Baumeister and John Tierney, explores fascinating studies on glucose levels in the blood affecting willpower: too little glucose and your willpower gets weaker. You need fuel in your body to make the best decisions.

Dr. Mattson's research, on the other hand, shows that consuming a near-constant stream of food appears to inhibit natural enzymes that protect our cells from aging.

Many nutritionists and health experts recommend eating small, healthy snacks, not only because this keeps your blood sugar stable, but also because it gives you another opportunity to eat fresh fruit and other healthy foods. And that may be the crux of the problem. The world is full of unhealthy snacks because people eat them, but the difference between reaching for an apple and reaching for a bag of Doritos is huge. None of the scientists I interviewed for this book, including Mattson, argued that a healthy, nutritious snack is a bad idea when you're really hungry and distracted by that hunger. Eating too many snacks, on the other hand, can get your body's hunger signals out of whack and lead to overeating and weight gain.

A middle-of-the-science approach looks something like this: don't snack unless you're hungry, but don't be afraid to stay hungry for a little while because at the very least, it will keep you sensitive to these important signals, and at best, it may help you age slower. Then, when you do reach for something to eat between meals, be sure it's nutritious.

Clock-Cheater Tip

A piece of fruit is an ideal snack. Other good grab-and-go snack ideas that have more nutrition than typical junk-food choices include celery sticks or apple slices with peanut butter, low- or nonfat yogurt or cottage cheese, a low-fat cheese stick paired with fruit or whole-grain crackers, a whole-wheat bagel or two whole-grain Fig Newtons, a cup of air-popped popcorn, a small box of raisins, or ¼ cup nuts.

Portion Proportion

Another reason people weigh more now is we eat larger portions today than we did 30 years ago, and it has made us fatter. In 1977, the average American ate 1,826 calories a day. By 2007, that figure had grown to 2,070 calories a day. An average person must consume about 3,500 excess calories to add 1 pound of weight, so eating about 250 extra calories a day can easily add a couple extra pounds a month.

One reason Americans eat larger portion sizes is that they eat out in restaurants much more than they used to, and in most cases, the amount of food served in restaurants is excessive. Renowned nutritionist Marion Nestle from New York University found that a "personal size" pizza at one restaurant in New York contained more than 2,000 calories—more than a typical woman should eat in a day. Most likely, no customer in the restaurant would ever guess the pizza contained so many calories!

Restaurants didn't used to serve so much food, but simple economics encouraged them to do it. Here's

> "A 'personal size' pizza at one restaurant in New York contained more than 2,000 calories—more than a typical woman should eat in a day."

why: in a chain restaurant, the highest cost of operating doesn't come from the food, it comes from paying people to cook and serve the food. So if it costs the restaurant the same thing to serve the food, they might as well serve larger meals they can charge more for. People buy the larger size because it seems like a better value.

Movie popcorn is a clear example. A large popcorn might cost just 50 cents more than a small even though it's twice the size, so ounce for ounce, it costs less, and customers see it as a better value. But the large popcorn still makes money because the extra popcorn in the large only costs the theater a few more cents. The psychology of good value tugs hard; even when someone doesn't necessarily want the extra food, they're inclined to buy the larger size because it's the best value. So the movie theater sells more large popcorns and makes more money.

This well-known principle of restaurant economics has compounded the psychological impact of larger portion sizes, which is that when we are given more food to eat, we eat more. As chain restaurants expanded around the country in the past 40 years, and we ate out more, we also ate more food because we were served bigger portions. And now we have an obesity crisis.

One of my favorite studies showing this effect was published in the journal *Obesity* in 2004. Researcher Barbara J. Rolls from Penn State University arranged for two different sizes of an entrée pasta to be served at a cafeteria on different days. One dish was 50 percent bigger than the other, but they were the same price. Consumers were unaware of the experiment, and when they were finished, the remaining food on their plates was discretely measured to determine how much they had eaten. Those who were served the larger portion sizes consumed 43 percent more food.

In questionnaires customers filled out after their meals, there was no difference in the way the large-entrée recipients and the small-entrée recipients rated the appropriateness of their portions. Both groups thought their portion was the right amount of food simply because that's what they were served!

Making the problem worse, those oversized portions have crept into our homes, too. People who eat out regularly have gotten used to eating more, making it harder to recognize what an appropriate-size meal should be. The psychology behind this phenomenon is also eye-opening. Several studies have documented that people who use larger plates serve themselves more food.

Another study found that people who used plates with a contrasting color from the food they were eating put more food on the plate. It turns out the contrast in colors plays a visual trick and makes the food look smaller on the plate than it actually is.

Because many people simply eat too much, part of the plan for aging well should include looking for ways to eat less. That may sound like dieting to you, but if your goal is to age well, take a longer view of losing weight.

Start with a few psychologically oriented solutions that can help cut down your caloric intake almost without trying. The known triggers of portion distortion can be used to make a few specific changes, such as buying smaller plates for entrées and desserts. You will serve yourself less food, but it won't seem like it.

Also, get an inexpensive set of different-colored plates (try Ikea or Pier 1 Imports) so you can try to match the color of the food you're serving to the plate color. It will make you eat less without even realizing it.

When you eat out, ask for a takeout container *when you get your food.* Before you eat, put some of your meal in the takeout container. It will have the same effect on your brain as walking away from a buffet: reduce the urge to eat it.

If you feel like having seconds (or reaching into that takeout container for another helping), try distracting yourself with a trip to the bathroom, a glass of water, or, best of all, a piece of fruit. The urge to eat more will usually pass. You'll soon get used to eating smaller portions!

Be sure, too, to eat slowly, paying attention to how good the food tastes and how much you're enjoying it. The hormonal signals that make you feel full can take a little while to register, so if you eat quickly, you may not feel full even if you've had enough—that's why after a big meal you may feel uncomfortably full 10 or 15 minutes after you're through. When you eat slowly, your body's natural satiety signals are more in sync with the rate at which you're eating.

This last point has been evident to me at home ever since I married Jim. As a result of a near-fatal choking incident in college, Jim always chews his food slowly and thoroughly before swallowing. Ironically, that near-death event may be contributing to his good health today because it's one reason he's never been an overeater. By taking longer to eat, he often feels full long before he feels the desire for seconds—plus he's always the last one finished. I have learned not to be offended when he doesn't want seconds of a meal I've worked hard to make!

Weight Loss and Aging

By purposefully eating just a little bit less—not by dieting, but by making slight changes to your environment and approach to food—you may well end up losing weight, which can lower your blood pressure and cholesterol, reverse or improve diabetes, improve your sleep, and more. Weight loss can also give you more energy and make you feel good about yourself, which are huge psychological benefits.

But does losing weight make you live longer—or at least stay healthier for longer? Population studies, in which larger numbers of subjects are followed over many years, suggest that overweight people do fare better over the long term if they shed some weight, especially if they're obese. But the real antiaging benefit comes from losing weight slowly and even better, from losing weight primarily by exercising more.

Clock-Cheater Tip
Maintaining your weight over your lifetime is associated with living longer, and one of the best strategies to keep your weight steady is to get on a bathroom scale every morning. That way, if you go up a pound, you can quickly adjust your diet to bring your weight back down in a couple days. Especially if you've worked hard to lose weight, use the scale to keep your weight from creeping back up. It's a lot easier to lose a pound as soon as you gain it than lose 10 pounds 2 months later!

"If you do not exercise while you are losing weight, what you are going to do is lose mostly muscle mass," explains Dr. Luigi Ferrucci, scientific director of the National Institute on Aging. "And so you are still contributing to the normal process of aging that tends to reduce lean body mass and increase fat mass."

Obese people have more reasons to lose weight than those who are just overweight because obesity is so harmful to health. But the average person who may need to lose 20 or 30 pounds, Ferrucci says, should consider losing weight only up to the age of about 65 or 70. Beyond that, he says, losing weight yields little or no benefit because it's stressful to the body and tends to accelerate the loss of muscle mass. Losing muscle in old age increases weakness and decreases activity, which in turn leads to more age-related complications. So at age 70, he advises to just maintain your weight but start moving around. If you're younger than 65, he says, lose weight slowly in conjunction with more exercise.

Of course, when it comes to aging well, and even mortality, there's no substitute for never having gained weight in the first place. "The people [who] do the best are the people who, at the age of 69 or 70, look very similar to the way they were at the age of 20," Ferrucci says.

That's pretty much true of Jim, who looks a lot like he did when he was 20, only thinner. Jim has lost 10 pounds over the past 5 years through gradual changes in his diet and by exercising more frequently. He never has overdone it with food, and his weight has stayed largely stable since college, fluctuating between 160 and 165 at 5 foot, 10 inches.

About 5 years ago, though, Jim's older brother died of cancer. His father died years ago of complications from diabetes. And other family members have a history of high blood pressure and heart disease. Given that Jim had a toddler and two grade-schoolers at home at the time, these facts were disconcerting. So he asked his internist, Dr. Elliot Aleskow, what he could do to improve his own health, and the doctor's answer was swift: "You're healthy, but you could lose ten pounds." He didn't make a big deal of it; he just told Jim to just eat a little bit less, exercise more, and lose weight slowly.

I vividly remember Jim coming home and saying, "There's no way I can lose ten pounds. My weight has been the same since I was in college." He had no intention of going on a diet, and you can't lose 10 pounds, he figured, if you don't go on a diet.

He was wrong.

How Jim Did It

In the past decade, Jim's diet has changed slowly but dramatically. Bit by bit, he has pared back the amount of food he eats and completely changed his consumption of whole grains, fruits, and vegetables.

My husband always enjoyed fruits and vegetables, but like many people, on most days, he didn't get the USDA's five recommended servings. Ten years ago, when he was in his mid-50s, he rarely had a fruit or vegetable at breakfast or lunch during the week, so on a good day, he'd get three servings at the most. But he has easily doubled his intake of these superfoods by adjusting his habits a little bit at a time. He's also more selective now about which fruits and vegetables he eats. "The darker the better," he likes to say.

Jim didn't set out to revamp his whole diet. Rather, he focused on one good habit gradually replacing a not-so-good habit, such as coming home from work and sitting down with a small pile of cheese puffs (organic, but still). This was such a common occurrence that we even had our own name for them, *pee-pah,* which is what our younger daughter, now 10, called them when she was a toddler and couldn't pronounce the words *cheese puffs*. In other words, they were around a lot. But not anymore—and we don't miss them. And that's just one of many things Jim has changed in his diet, painlessly. The story of how cheese puffs disappeared from our house, and how Jim made many other changes to his diet, offers a great model for anyone who wants to ditch bad dietary habits and add good new ones.

The result of this gradual, easy transformation has been that Jim now weighs 150 pounds, even though up until 5 years ago, he had never in his adult life weighed less than 160 pounds. Also interesting to note is that in the past 5 years—from age 58 to 63—Jim has shown almost no visible signs of aging, especially in his skin and hair, but also in his energy level and overall health. Is there a relationship between his lack of aging and his much higher consumption of vitamins, minerals, fiber, and antioxidants? The science suggests there is.

> "Is there a relationship between his lack of aging and his much higher consumption of vitamins, minerals, fiber, and antioxidants? The science suggests there is."

Slow Change

It wasn't really intentional when Jim started eating more vegetables. He has always liked green vegetables, even some that get a bad rep, like brussels sprouts. But when I went into early labor with our first child, who is now a young teenager, I was put on strict bed rest for 6 weeks. All of a sudden, Jim was thrown into doing all the household duties, including grocery shopping, with no help. Every week he would take off to do a major run to the supermarket on Sunday and then come into the living room with great fanfare and show me, as I lay on the couch, the great meals he planned to make that week.

Every week he came home with brussels sprouts. Mind you, I have always liked these much-maligned little veggie balls, thanks to my father's wonderful, fresh method of cooking them, which I'll share later in the book. But 6 weeks in a row was a bit much.

That was a turning point for Jim, though, because since we'd gotten married he had exercised little control over what we ate; I generally do the shopping and cooking, and he does the dishes, which has worked for us. I like cooking, and he likes to crank up the music in the kitchen while he cleans up.

During the time I was on bed rest, though, Jim made us simple, light meals that showcased the freshness of the vegetables. Guided by his cooking skills, pretty much everything was raw (salad, tomatoes), steamed (asparagus, broccoli), or blanched (green beans, brussels sprouts) and featured few sauces or dishes to wash. His comfort zone in the kitchen didn't extend much beyond a simple sautéed chicken breast or broiled piece of fish, either. So every night dinner was a bit of lean protein and half a plate of vegetables—significantly simpler than the dinners I was used to preparing, which tended to involve a good deal more actual "cooking." I longed for some risotto, pasta, sauces, and spices, but I really appreciated his hard work, so what could I say?

Our new nightly menu may have been a product of necessity—and Jim's admittedly limited time and cooking experience—but he started saying he liked the way it made him feel: energetic and not overly full. He called it "eating clean" (even as he followed these healthy foods with one too many cookies!). Indeed, we both began to feel better, although lying on the couch 8 months pregnant doesn't do anyone's appetite or energy any good. But after the baby was born and I was back on my feet and cooking again, I started making more meals like Jim's: quick, simple, and largely unadorned. It worked with our new baby-induced time constraints, it felt good, and Jim was able to participate more in preparing our meals.

We soon realized, though, that Jim's idea of a vegetable had almost always been something green, whereas I ventured more into other colors, such as yellow corn, red tomatoes, and red cabbage, while also serving grains such as rice and polenta. But in his 6 weeks as house chef, Jim had grown attached to having a green vegetable every night, so we adapted, and he began making a salad whenever we weren't having something green on our plates. Ironically, we had both grown up with a salad on the dinner table with every meal but had both fallen out of that regular habit.

The result of this collaboration is that most nights we ended up having two vegetables with dinner, but it was a small change that quickly became a regular routine and definitely upped our intake of antioxidant-rich vegetables.

More recently, Jim has continued to influence our vegetable selections more purposefully based on their healthfulness. When he reads something about an especially nutritious vegetable, he'll bring it home the next time he does the grocery shopping. That has led to terrific dinners with more variety, such as sautéed spinach, baked sweet potatoes, braised bok choy, and stir-fried cabbage.

> "Most nights we ended up having two vegetables with dinner, but it was a small change that quickly became a regular routine and definitely upped our intake of antioxidant-rich vegetables."

Thankfully, I have one of the best cookbooks ever written to help cook any kind of vegetable: *The Victory Garden Cookbook* by Marian Morash. It was one of my father's favorites, and he gave it to me and my sister for Christmas many years ago. It's arranged alphabetically and contains great details about how countless vegetables are grown, how to choose a good one, and myriad cooking techniques and delicious and unexpected recipes. My copy is dog-eared and stained. I love it.

We also began looking for inspiration from professionals. At a delightful restaurant in Washington called Kafe Leopold, we fell in love with the chopped kale salad, which we shared one weekend day at lunchtime. We had never eaten kale raw, but this salad was so good, we began adding it to our salads at home now and then, especially if we found small and tender baby kale at the store. Kale (baby leaves or chopped-up mature ones) makes a meaty and delicious salad that's packed with vitamins and antioxidants. It can also handle a robust dressing, such as something sweet or spicy.

A Fruitful Effort

But perhaps the biggest change in Jim's diet has been in the past 5 years, as he has gradually increased the amount of fruit he eats. Ten years ago, the only time he consistently ate fruit, besides fresh orange juice with breakfast every day, was on the weekends, when we might have strawberries with our pancakes on Sunday mornings, or if apples or grapes were around at lunchtime. Now he eats large portions of fruit at least twice a day, every day, even at work.

But this change didn't begin deliberately, and it wasn't quick: it took a year or two to fall into the routine of eating this way. This gradualness made the change hardly noticeable, so Jim never missed the "old" foods he used to eat regularly.

Jim's increased fruit consumption started when the youngest of our three children (now 8) was a toddler. I have fed our children fresh fruit with every meal and snack since they started eating solid food. As they would tell you, it's simply non-negotiable in our house! But it's one thing to do this when they're little and have little stomachs; it's another thing entirely when they're growing like weeds and plowing through the entire contents of the refrigerator at an alarming pace. So keeping up with this five-fruits-a-day routine became not only time-consuming, but also expensive: fruit at breakfast, fruit at snacktime for the kids who were home, fruit at lunch, fruit after school, and fruit at dinner. Times three. Yikes.

To make it possible, I started going to Costco every couple weeks and buying larger quantities of fresh fruit, cutting it up, and storing it in plastic containers so there would always be easy access to cut fruit in the fridge. It was a quick, inexpensive way to keep this healthy habit going as the kids got bigger.

And then Jim started stealing our fruit.

The thievery began after he read an article about the healthy nutrients in watermelon, a fruit you might normally assume was relatively nutrition free. It is not. Watermelon is not only high in vitamins C, B_6, and A, it also contains potassium, fiber, and important amino acids. Plus, watermelon has only 30 calories in about 1 cup fruit!

Clock-Cheater Tip

Watermelon contains vitamins A, C, B_6, and thiamin, and also has more of the powerful antioxidant lycopene than tomatoes. What's more, according to Dr. Bahram H. Arjmandi, chair of the department of Nutrition, Food, and Exercise Sciences at Florida State University, it's the richest edible source of the amino acid L-cytrilline. In the body, this compound is transformed into nitric oxide, which helps regulate the health of the vascular system and blood pressure. "Watermelon reduces both brachial and aortic blood pressure," says Arjmandi, whose latest study on the health effects of watermelon was published in 2012 in the *American Journal of Hypertension*.

As I've said, Jim had often come home from work and sat down with a bag of cheese puffs. Running a busy law practice takes a toll on him during the day, so when he gets home, he wants a little pick-me-up before getting into gear with the children or whatever else is going on. Around the time he read the article on watermelon, he opened the refrigerator and noticed a container of cut watermelon, with all its antioxidants and vitamin C, staring him in the face. So he took it out and started eating. Because it was summertime, we had a lot of watermelon around, so Jim was eating it regularly, and pretty soon he found he wasn't eating as many cheese puffs. When there wasn't any watermelon in the fridge, he began eating any other cut or washed fruit he might find: cantaloupe, grapes, berries, pineapple. Without planning it, his mid-evening, predinner consumption of fruit became something he loved to do and gradually replaced the less-healthy snacks he used to eat.

When he read another article about the high nutrition content of pistachio nuts, which he has always loved, that put the cheese puffs on the chopping block for good. It just didn't seem right to eat all this healthy fruit and follow it up with junk food. Pistachios, though, contain many healthy compounds and are high in various vitamins, minerals, and fiber. In one study published in *The American Journal of Clinical Nutrition,* a diet rich in pistachio nuts was found to lower levels of "bad" cholesterol, which is a risk factor for cardiovascular disease.

Now, Jim's daily snack isn't cheese puffs, it's just fruit and occasionally a handful (or two!) of pistachio nuts. The frequent buy-one-get-one-free deals on berries at the supermarket are now a magnet for me: buy one for Jim, get one for the rest of us!

In this gradual, almost accidental way, Jim dramatically increased his intake of antiaging vitamins, fiber, and antioxidants and has kept it there for about 3 years now. I can't imagine he'll ever go back: the transition was not only painless, it has been a joy. Without a doubt, he feels healthier than he ever has and his skin looks even smoother and brighter than it used to.

> "Without planning it, his mid-evening, predinner consumption of fruit became something he loved to do and gradually replaced the less-healthy snacks he used to eat."

Targeting Meals

As Jim began to feel better, he became more mindful of his food choices—and along the way, he targeted what he ate for breakfast, which, for years, was a piece of white toast with jam on it, orange juice, and a cup of tea. Protein? Nope. Fiber? Nope. Antioxidants? Nope. Only his orange juice had some nutritional value—but also a lot of sugar.

The first thing he did was cut back to half a piece of toast and added yogurt for the protein. For a long time, he ate plain yogurt with honey or a serving-size container of fruit yogurt. It didn't take long to notice that the added protein at breakfast kept him going longer through the morning. That positive effect turned him, over the course of a few months, from someone who almost never ate yogurt into a true yogurt fan.

Excited by the positive impact this simple—and delicious—change had been, Jim started experimenting with the rest of breakfast to see if he could get an even better energy boost through the morning. He began buying different kinds of whole-grain cereals to try, starting with Kashi GOLEAN, which he liked and was easily available at the supermarkets. But it was hard to make this transition quickly, and he missed his toast. So he would alternate, while continuing to look for other cereals that satisfied him. Sometimes he would comment that he liked the way one cereal tasted, but it got soggy. Or he liked the texture of another but it was too sweet.

Clock-Cheater Tip

It was worth the effort, though, when you consider the impact that just a single bowl of whole-grain cereal can make to your long-term health—and possibly your lifespan. In a large study of 21,000 people followed over 19 years as part of the Physician's Health Study, researchers from Harvard reported in 2007 that people who ate just one bowl of whole-grain cereal every morning lowered their risk of heart failure by 29 percent, even excluding the effect of exercise, family history, and diet, among other things.

Then he hit on the idea of mixing them, and that was the answer. He began with two or three, but his mixture has grown more complex. Now each morning he routinely combines four to six different kinds of whole-grain cereals. He still tries new things, but he's a big reader of labels, looking for cereals with whole grains, plenty of protein, and not a lot of sugar. Usually, his mix includes Grape-Nuts; one or another Kashi cereal; Special K Protein Plus flakes or Nature's Path Heritage Flakes; and some combination of granola, muesli, or rolled oats. He tops it off with some wheat germ and raisins or a few walnuts for the omega-3 fatty acids.

I tease him as he does this routine in the morning, but he enjoys the creativity of preparing his cereal, and he likes to mix it up a little every day. For all that effort, he doesn't eat a huge bowl of cereal—maybe $3/4$ cup, with skim milk. But wow, does it pay off: he's less hungry and has more energy throughout the day, plus all those vitamins, minerals, and fiber are helping keep his cells happy and youthful.

"I used to get hungry by 10 or 11, and by noon I was ready to go out and buy lunch," he said. "Now I find I sometimes don't even get hungry."

Clock-Cheater Tip

You don't have to be tied to one cereal in your bowl. If you love Corn Flakes but wish it were more nutritious, add some whole-grain oat cereal, a few walnuts, and some strawberries, or whatever you find that has plenty of whole grains and not a lot of sugar. Experiment until you find a delicious mix you love that does a better job of nourishing your cells and keeping them young.

On a recent family trip to the beach, Jim offered some of his cereal concoction to my mother, who is 84 and lives near us. She had it every morning and loved it, so now he makes it for her regularly!

The final change he made to breakfast came a few years ago when he, like so many people, fell in love with Greek yogurt. He eats Chobani yogurt every morning now, marveling that it could have so much protein, no cholesterol, and (in most flavors) no fat—yet still taste so good. He has stuck with this breakfast for 2 or 3 years now and looks forward to it every morning.

The benefits of changing his breakfast routine were so startling that Jim began looking for other ways to get whole grains into his diet. I generally do the grocery shopping, and I must have tried seven or eight different whole-wheat breads before I found one we all like—a double-protein whole-wheat bread made by Arnold. I've ruined more batches of brown rice than I care to admit (it's a little tricky to cook, in my opinion), so I finally began buying pouches of frozen brown rice at Trader Joe's. It's quick and easy to prepare and delicious when drizzled with a touch of healthful canola oil and sprinkled with a little salt and pepper. But those additions are optional. We still eat white rice on occasion, but hardly ever and no one in our family misses it.

In 2011, the government adjusted its dietary guidelines away from the confusing food pyramid to the much more meaningful My Plate guide, which basically illustrates exactly the way we eat. If everything we ate for dinner fit on one plate, TV-dinner style, half the plate would be fruits and vegetables, a small portion would be lean protein, and another small portion, on many nights, would be some sort of whole grain or other healthy starch, such as a sweet potato.

> "The benefits of changing his breakfast routine were so startling that Jim began looking for other ways to get whole grains into his diet."

Now Jim's dietary changes have gradually crept into his workplace. Jim used to buy lunch every day, usually a sandwich, and bring it back to the office to eat at his desk while reading the newspaper—a necessary and much-appreciated break in the middle of a hectic day. But "I would often feel too full, and it was harder to get my energy back for work as quickly as I needed to," he says.

He started getting soup and half a sandwich but then noticed containers of mixed fruit at his usual lunch spot, so he decided to try that instead of soup. After a few days, he found the adjustment made him more productive right after lunch because he wasn't as tired, so he stuck with it. He doesn't miss the soup. But the extension of his fruit-eating habit has been another step on the road to greater consumption of antioxidants, while also reducing the number of calories he eats. Now he buys a large container of fruit, eats half of it, and puts the rest in the refrigerator to eat for lunch the next day. Instead of eating a whole sandwich with his fruit, he ate half a sandwich and added a few pretzels—maybe not a health food, but it has been another change that has cut his overall calorie intake.

And finally, he now saves several hundred calories a week by not eating a whole bag of peanut M&M's after lunch, which he had done every day since I'd known him. After Halloween a few years ago, Jim grabbed a few leftover trick-or-treat-size baggies of peanut M&M's from the candy bowl and took them to the office to eat after lunch.

They were smaller, "but I can't bring myself to open another bag. It just feels like too much," he said at the time. So when the little bags were about to run out, I suggested we count the number of M&Ms in the small bags versus a regular bag. It turned out to be 9 or 10, almost exactly half of what's in the regular bag. So he now counts out 9 or 10 M&M's for his after-lunch treat.

These purposeful changes made a big difference in Jim's weight. The weight loss was so gradual, I didn't notice it on him, and he didn't really notice it on the scale. But every once in a while he would put on an article of clothing he hadn't worn in a while and notice that it fit better or looked better. Over the past 3 years, he has lost those 10 pounds he said he'd never be able to lose. And he did it without going on a diet. Yes, he counted M&M's, but he doesn't view it as deprivation; he views it as smart and effective.

The takeaway message is that changing your diet can be on your terms. You don't need to eat what someone else tells you to eat. Figure out what you like, and come up with a way to eat less of it. Or find something you like you know is healthy and figure out a way to eat it more often, by taking it to work, for example. Don't worry about the time frame when it comes to changing your diet; it may take a while to find things you enjoy, but it's worth it, and the time doesn't matter as much as the fact that you're working toward getting there. Every step you take to improve makes you feel a little bit better and makes you want to improve more. Eventually, it'll add up to feeling better, looking younger, and aging more slowly.

Clock-Cheater Tip

If you want to start eating less but you have a hard time dieting, give yourself a longer time frame. Set a goal of reducing one part of your diet every couple weeks by just a little bit, and give yourself a chance to get used to it. When you do, pick something else. After a year, you'll have made a noticeable dent in what you eat, and it won't feel like a diet. The next year, you can either keep going, or depending on how much you've reduced your calories, watch the weight slowly come off.

It's hard to overstate the impact my husband's new dietary habits have on his energy level, looks, and health. Among other things, he hasn't had a cold in 3 years.

Incorporating these healthful changes means Jim can still eat the things he wants to without worry, including pretzels, M&M's, a glass of wine with dinner every night, cookies for dessert, and of course the occasional extra treat, such as ice cream with the kids.

Jim is not a health-food nut or a nutrition junkie. He's just a regular guy who took his time to find a healthier choice he liked and could stick to. And it has had an amazing effect on how he's aging. It's a cliché, but truly, if he can do it, anyone can.

Supplement Science

Jim's evolving and improving nutrition habits have clearly helped him fight the effects of aging, but I wouldn't be giving the complete picture without mentioning that he's been taking regular vitamin E supplements, 200 international units (IU) a day, for 40 years.

Yes, *every day*.

The scientists I spoke to about Jim spent some obvious time trying to figure out how to respond when I told them about the vitamin E supplements my husband takes. Why? Because vitamin E is controversial. Several recent high-profile clinical trials involving vitamin E have found either no benefit from the supplement or possible harmful effects.

There's a tremendous amount of published research on vitamin E, and more research is going on all the time, in animals and in humans. Many of these studies have positive outcomes, while others are inconclusive or somewhat negative. For example, a study published in the *Journal of the American Medical Association* in 2012 showed taking 400 IU a day (roughly 270 milligrams natural vitamin E) could raise a man's risk of prostate cancer. Yet an earlier study of 29,000 Finnish men, all of whom were smokers, found a significant decrease in the risk of prostate cancer from taking vitamin E.

Different Types of Vitamin E

Vitamin E comes in numerous forms, but alpha-tocopherol is the only one that stays in the blood, so federal recommendations refer only to alpha-tocopherol. Alpha-tocopherol can come from natural sources (derived from plants) or from synthetic sources (made in a lab). The molecular structure of natural vitamin E is more easily used in the body, so you need a smaller dose. They are labeled differently—natural vitamin E is *d*-alpha-tocopherol while synthetic is *dl*-alpha-tocopherol—so be sure to pay attention to the label.

Now much of the scientific community doesn't know what to say about a vitamin that seems to hold so much promise. Vitamin E is one of the most powerful antioxidants in nature, and it plays important roles in keeping our cells functioning normally and protecting them from many of the conditions that commonly appear as we age. In simple terms, vitamin E helps protect fatty structures in the body, including cell membranes, brain tissue, and cholesterol (both the HDL "good" kind and the LDL "bad" kind). Fatty tissues in the body are easily damaged when bombarded by free radicals, and vitamin E, because it's fat-soluble, helps limit this oxidation and keep those structures and molecules intact.

Among others, vitamin E has these positive effects:

- Increases vasodilation—the relaxing of the smooth muscles inside the walls of large veins, arteries, and other blood vessels, widening them for improved blood flow.
- Boosts molecules and enzymes involved in immunity response.
- Limits cognitive decline and inhibits the formation of cataracts.
- Helps prevent blood clots, much the way aspirin does.

Measuring Vitamins

Vitamins and minerals are measured differently depending on the source and purpose. For example, vitamin E is measured both in international units (IU) and milligrams. An IU is a measurement of *biological activity,* the size of which is decided by consensus of the scientific community. Milligrams are a measurement of *quantity.* The recommended daily intake (RDI) for vitamins and minerals are given in measurements of quantity, usually milligrams (one-thousandth gram) or micrograms (one-millionth gram). Supplements are measured in IU. Vitamins have different conversion rates. For vitamin D, 1 microgram equals 40 IU. For vitamin E, 1 milligram equals 1.49 IU natural vitamin E and 2.22 milligrams synthetic vitamin E. To get the recommended 15 milligrams of vitamin E, you need 22.4 IU natural vitamin E or 33.3 IU synthetic vitamin E.

Other positive effects have also been observed in lab animals and humans taking vitamin E, so not surprisingly, scientists remain very excited about the potential role of vitamin E in healthy aging. Researchers at The Ohio State University, for example, announced in 2013 that they had identified a previously unknown anti-cancer molecule in a particular form of Vitamin E (called gamma tocopherol) that suppressed tumor growth in mice. The discovery could lead to a new type of nontoxic cancer drug.

Still, supplements should be approached with caution, and scientists recommend that Americans focus on getting their recommended 15 milligrams a day of vitamin E from vegetable oils, nuts, whole grains, and leafy greens. (By contrast, many of the big vitamin E studies are using very large doses of vitamin E, up to 600 or 800 IU a day, which could be causing other harmful side effects, experts say.)

Dr. Maret Traber, nutritional biochemist at the Linus Pauling Institute at the University of Oregon, is one of the world's top vitamin E scientists. She was on the panel of experts who came up with the Institute of Medicine's 2000 recommendation to the government for daily intake of vitamin E. She is now conducting more research for future intake recommendations, should there be a revision.

Traber is not dismissive of the studies that have found vitamin E to be harmful or neutral, but she cautions that the results of complex studies can sometimes be wrong for unknown reasons, or give mixed signals that can be interpreted incorrectly.

"There's something called the Women's Health Study that was run out of Harvard where they gave women 45 years and older 600 IUs of vitamin E every other day for 10 years," Traber says. "The purpose of this experiment was to ask, 'Does vitamin E prevent heart disease in otherwise healthy women?' Their global answer was 'no'—oops, except for in the women who were 65 and older, there is a 50 percent decrease in cardiovascular disease."

Clock-Cheater Tip

Find excellent, easy-to-understand scientific and technical information on dozens of vitamins, minerals, and supplements on the NIH's Office of Dietary Supplements website, ndb.nal.usda.gov.

If possible, Dr. Traber says healthy individuals should try to get more vitamin E in their diets from fortified cereals, whole grains, healthy oils, and certain fruits and vegetables, rather than from supplements. But truthfully, it's hard to get enough in your diet.

"96 percent of American women and 90 percent of American men don't meet the requirements for vitamin E," she says. Even people who eat lots of fruits, vegetables, and nuts generally have a hard time meeting the requirement because they would have to eat more broccoli, spinach, or almonds than anyone would want to. Given that, Jim's supplements make some sense, Traber says. It's more than he needs, even if the excess is excreted harmlessly by the liver. "Maybe once a week is good enough," she says.

Aside from vitamin E, most of the nutritionists and scientists I spoke with say that people who don't eat well should take a standard multivitamin. But few were willing to advise taking other supplements over getting the right nutrition from food because food sources of vitamins come in the right form and are easy for your body to absorb.

Dietary Sources of Vitamin E

According to the USDA, good sources of vitamin E include almonds (1 ounce = 6.8 milligrams); avocados (1 medium = 3 milligrams); broccoli ($\frac{1}{2}$ cup = 1.2 milligrams); kiwifruit (1 medium = 1.1 milligrams); peanut butter (2 tablespoons = 2.9 milligrams); sunflower seeds (1 ounce = 7.4 milligrams); steamed spinach ($\frac{1}{2}$ cup = 1.9 milligrams); tomato spaghetti sauce (1 cup = 5.5 milligrams); and vegetable oils such as grapeseed, sunflower, or safflower (1 tablespoon = 6 to 10 milligrams). You can find the nutrient content of many foods, sorted by nutrient, online at nal.usda.gov/fnic/foodcomp/Data. Click the Nutrients List link.

Obviously, supplementation is something you need to discuss with your doctor. But Dr. Luigi Ferrucci of the National Institute on Aging summed up his view of supplementation this way:

"I think that we have good data only for omega-3 fatty acids and vitamin D. Everything else is highly questionable," he says. "We know that vitamin D in women actually prevents fractures and is associated with maintenance of bone density. And we know that people [who] take high doses of omega-3 fatty acids, both in terms of diet, a fish-based diet, or supplementation, tend to have lower risk of sudden death and lowered risk of cardiovascular disease. We know that because every study ever done always showed that. For the others, the results are so inconsistent that nobody is really willing to give a recommendation."

Part 3

Moving Matters

The Pathways
Less Traveled

If there's one question most people hate to be asked during a physical, it's this: "How much do you exercise?"

"I, uhhh, try to get to the gym most weeks but, uh, you know, it's just been really hard lately because I've been so busy at work ...."

If this sounds familiar, you're not alone. I've been guilty myself. According to the Centers for Disease Control (CDC), only *8 percent* of Americans get the recommended amount of exercise a week—defined as roughly 30 minutes of moderately intense activity a day, such as brisk walking, golfing with no cart, mowing the lawn, cleaning the house, playing racket sports, or leisurely canoeing.

That the CDC includes "leisurely canoeing" as one of its possible daily activity should not detract from the true message that our exercise rates are horrifyingly low.

Why horrifying? Because when it comes to keeping the human body in good form through the years, exercise is second only to nutrition in effectiveness. What scientists have discovered recently, however, is how much exercise does for you on the inside. Exercise does your body good—in your cells—in ways you can't see and may not even feel, but that make a dramatic difference to your health over the years.

Everyone knows, generally speaking, that exercise is good for you. It makes you fit, helps your heart, lifts your mood, keeps your weight down, curbs your appetite, and gives you more energy. When done regularly, it can make you look better, reduce anxiety, ease depression, help you sleep, and create more satisfaction with your life. In short, it can make you happy.

So why is it that 92 percent of us don't do it? "The number one reason people give for not being active is lack of time," explains Dr. David C. Nieman, director of the Human Performance Laboratory at Appalachian State University in North Carolina. Nieman, when he's not in the lab investigating exercise physiology and its relationship to human health, teaches three college courses, regularly publishes articles in scientific journals, has written nine books, and sits on various editorial and medical boards. He has also run 58 marathons and ultra-marathons.

That should make it pretty clear that lack of time, although it might be part of the problem, is not the true reason people don't exercise. After all, if Nieman can find the time to train for and run 58 marathons, the rest of us can squeeze in 30 minutes of table tennis every day (yes, that's also on the CDC's list of moderate-intensity exercise), along with some sit-ups and push-ups.

We don't do it, though, because it's hard—harder, anyway, than sinking into the couch with a drink at the end of a long day. And most people, when given a choice, will choose the activity that feels better at that moment. If exercising felt the same as relaxing right off the bat, we would all run marathons like Nieman. It's the same equation that makes us fat: if an apple tasted the same as a cupcake, we would all be thin.

Early humans, of course, exercised *a lot* because there was all that hunting and gathering to do. But even back then, 100,000 years ago, in the few periods when we didn't have to exert ourselves just to survive, we rested to save our energy. Now, thanks to the rise of industrialized society, where many people don't have to be active every day, we avoid it because we can. Plus it's easy to do nothing: our big brains blessed us with the capability to create pleasurable, restful activities in place of less-enjoyable, more-arduous ones. The car is a good example.

> "Our big brains blessed us with the capability to create pleasurable, restful activities in place of less-enjoyable, more-arduous ones."

But there's a big problem with that. Once your body gets deconditioned, your heart gets a little weaker and your muscles get a little smaller. That makes exercise feel even harder. What you end up with, in many people, is a condition that rhymes with *hazy*. When you've reached that point, it takes a really long time to force yourself to exercise. So naturally, no one has time to do it.

Yet 8 percent of people do exercise, so what's the difference between them and the rhymes-with-*hazy* people? The difference is having a reason to exercise. Some people have coaches or friends who push them to get moving. Others exercise because their health—or life—depends on it. But the vast majority of people, Nieman says, exercise because they like the way it makes them feel. There's a leap there, of course, because you can't get to the point that exercise makes you feel good until you get past the point that exercise *doesn't* feel good.

What you need is a really good reason to exercise and a way to do it that doesn't hurt.

Thanks to the hard work being done by scientists like Dr. Nieman, who have been gradually unlocking the secrets of exercise's effects on the human body, here are three good reasons you haven't heard before why you should get off the couch and into that canoe (metaphorically speaking, of course):

1. Scientists have proven that exercise slows down—and even reverses—the aging process.
2. You don't have to do very much exercise, or do it very strenuously, to get antiaging benefits.
3. No kidding.

The interplay of exercise and aging is astonishingly complex, so there's a lot that's unknown. But the scientific understanding of the benefits of exercise has advanced tremendously in recent years. There's now a dramatic body of evidence that moderate exercise—the kind that feels good right from the start—activates a hidden system of defense and renewal that can, quite simply, turn back the clock.

How does this work? By moving around with just medium effort, even in 10-minute bursts (but at least 10 minutes, Nieman says), you set in motion a cascade of reactions inside your cells that have positive effects. For example, exercise triggers the release of enzymes that turn on genes, trigger proteins, and stimulate the brain to generate new neurons. In other words, you walk, you breathe a little harder, and a few cellular steps later, your brain grows. It happens microscopically, of course, but it adds up.

> "There's now a dramatic body of evidence that moderate exercise—the kind that feels good right from the start—activates a hidden system of defense and renewal that can, quite simply, turn back the clock."

Unfortunately, the opposite is also true. If you don't walk, and you don't ever breathe hard, your brain shrinks. Literally. It's not detectable in a day or a week or a month, of course, but over the years, a few neurons at a time, this process plays a critical role in the size and activity of your brain and, therefore, in your mental and physical health.

This kind of sequential response in your cells is known as a *pathway*. Pathways in which enzymes, proteins, genes, amino acids, and hormones all work together are responsible for nearly every aspect of how your body lives, moves, and dies. Unfortunately, these beneficial pathways that are triggered by exercise are sitting dormant in most of us, and increasingly so as we age.

This is a shame, because we don't start out that way. Most kids love to run around and be physical. Then, in school, they get exercise through physical education, recess, and sports. But unless it comes from the parents, most children aren't taught the value of exercise simply for exercise's sake. So when they grow up and there's no recess and no way to play football, they're suddenly faced with that same easy but fateful choice: the sofa or the StairMaster. The sofa usually wins.

"What we need to focus our school policy on is sports we can do as we get older, going for a run or a walk, or how you set up a little gym or circuit set and what can you do with your partner," says Dr. Mark Tarnopolsky, professor and cell biologist at McMaster University in Hamilton, Ontario, Canada, who studies exercise extensively. "Those are the activities you need to learn, because if you don't learn them in school, you don't know how to do them later on. Once you get out of shape it's a bear to get back in shape."

The result of this collective lack of exercise—and the lack of will on the part of policymakers to make exercise mandatory in schools—will be a wave of illness, dementia, disease, and early death 40 years from now, when there will be 88 million people in this country age 65 and older, most of whom never knew the *real* reasons why they should have exercised and eaten right.

"It never gets translated to the policymakers. I think all they care about is the next four years," Tarnopolsky says. "We're going to be in big trouble when we have many more older adults. The data is there. It's objective. It's not, 'oh, I believe this and it's some sort of religion.' It's real stuff. You can choose to take it, or ignore it."

This is how scientists who study aging tend to view the future, based on their very real—and alarming—research. But as much as scientists like Dr. Tarnopolsky know about how much exercise can do to prevent ill health in one's later years, that message doesn't get out there: exercise is still most often viewed—and sold—primarily as a way to get a sexy body. That certainly prompts plenty of people to start exercise programs every year, which is good. But for most people, that lofty result remains unattainable, so they give up because what's the point? They knock themselves out for a month and then think, *If I'm not going to look any different, why should I keep killing myself on the treadmill?*

> "The best reason to exercise is not to look hot now, but to remain healthy, pain free, mentally sharp, and energetic, now and into your twilight years. It's the original preventive medicine."

What not enough people know—really, truly understand—is just how important exercise is for health, vitality, and aging. The best reason to exercise is not to look hot now, but to remain healthy, pain free, mentally sharp, and energetic, now and into your twilight years. It's the original preventive medicine.

If you knew what scientists know about how exercise prevents age-related decline, you'd probably get off the couch. So in this chapter and next, you learn about the science of exercise and what it really does for you (and no, I'm not talking about washboard abs), along with the best way to do it. But before we get to that, there are three important points to remember about exercising to age well:

- It takes less exercise to age well than it does to get physically fit.
- It's never too late to benefit from exercise.
- You can build up slowly over many years because the effects are cumulative.

That tidal wave of Alzheimer's disease, disability, and depression that's coming down the pike? Exercise is your ticket off the island.

Of Mice and Muscles

The benefits of exercise, scientists like to say, are *multifactorial*. In other words, exercise does a lot of good in a lot of ways. But luckily, scientists aren't content to leave it at that, so new information keeps pouring in about the specific ways exercise helps you.

"We're used to reducing things down to one pathway, x, y, or z, and analyzing the heck out of it," says exercise scientist Tarnopolsky. That's exactly what he does: Tarnopolsky and a team of researchers investigate the effect of exercise on muscle health and a variety of degenerative conditions, including aging.

Dr. Tarnopolsky's research on people and animals has focused largely on one mechanism in the aging process: the mitochondria. These are the tiny structures inside your cells that are the power plants for your body, turning your food into energy your cells can use. One thing that happens during aging is that over time, your mitochondria are damaged by oxidative stress (when destructive free radicals spill out of the mitochondria during the energy-making process). When mitochondria are damaged, they don't produce as much energy, so more of the calories you consume are stored as fat rather than turned into fuel. Eventually, malfunctioning mitochondria lead to cell senescence or cell death, both of which contribute to aging and decreased tissue function, and can lead to cancer.

Tarnopolsky wondered if exercise is so beneficial because it does something magical to the mitochondria. He started with a colony of mice he had bred with a specific genetic mutation that prevented their mitochondria from being repaired after damage from oxidative stress—a condition that leads to drastically premature aging in the mice. Then he divided the colony into two groups—one group that lived normal lab lives with no exercise, and another that exercised on a wheel for 45 minutes three times a week from age 3 months to age 8 months.

At the end of that time, the mice that didn't exercise were victims of their decaying mitochondria: they were old-looking and decrepit, with thinning fur, brain atrophy, hearing loss, muscle shrinkage, anemia, smaller gonads, and overall weakness. The genetically identical exercised mice, however, were completely normal, with the youthful looks, energy, and health of normal 8-month-old mice.

"We found, essentially, nearly 100 percent protection in the exercisers," Tarnopolsky says.

So what did the exercise do? It activated a pathway that increased production of a protein, that regulated a set of genes, that improved the function of the mitochondria. And lucky for the mice, it also activated a previously unidentified system that was able to *repair* the mitochondria, even though the mice had been bred without the only gene known to control mitochondria repair. Dr. Tarnopolsky's group is doing more work to figure out exactly how that worked.

Recent research has also shown that exercise doesn't just help repair mitochondria, it also can generate new mitochondria, especially in muscles. This is particularly important in delaying aging because one of the most common conditions that affects older Americans is the gradual loss of muscle mass. Over the years, cumulative oxidative stress and mitochondrial damage break down the muscle tissue. People who don't exercise start losing muscle mass at the rate of about 1 percent per year, beginning in the fourth decade of life. Eventually, it leads to loss of mobility and independence, which in turn leads to even less activity and even greater vulnerability to disease. If there were a way to increase the number and function of mitochondria in the muscle, it would have huge implications for maintaining movement and health through the years.

Exercise, Tarnopolsky has shown, does just that.

Tarnopolsky did experiments on about 60 adults ranging in age from 65 to 86, putting them through a moderate strength-training program on their legs for 4 to 6 months. Biopsies of their leg muscles taken before and after the program showed that mitochondria production in their leg muscles increased "very significantly," he said, and the subjects reported much greater mobility and muscle strength.

Other startling exercise research has been conducted by biochemist Simon Melov at the Buck Institute for Research on Aging in California. In one experiment, groups of healthy, moderately active (but not athletic) younger and older adults were both put through hour-long resistance-training programs in a gym twice a week. The researchers took tissue samples from the thigh muscles of the participants and compared the two age groups. The older adults, with an average age of 70, began the program with 59 percent less leg strength than the younger group, which had an average age of 21. By the end of the program, that difference was only 38 percent.

> "People who don't exercise start losing muscle mass at the rate of about 1 percent per year, beginning in the fourth decade of life."

An even more dramatic improvement was seen on the genetic level, when the scientists looked inside the muscle cells of the two groups. "Following exercise training, the [genetic] signature of aging was markedly reversed ... to that of younger levels," the study explains.

The exercise had benefitted both groups, but it had benefitted the older group much more. Quite simply, exercise had reversed the aging process.

Age Better with Exercise

Scientists around the world are researching the effect of exercise on every aspect of aging. There's something about exercise that causes systemic improvements in health, affecting far more than the systems you'd naturally expect to improve with exercise, such as the cardiovascular system. To figure out how exercise does this, researchers are looking at the benefits of physical activity at the cellular level. They have found that exercise does quite a few things:

- Protects telomeres
- Augments your immune system
- Reduces oxidative stress
- Boosts metabolism
- Increases brain size
- Enhances your sleep
- Helps regulate hunger

Let's look at each in detail.

Exercise Protects Telomeres

Remember the little caps on the ends of your chromosomes that protect your DNA from damage when cells divide? These telomeres shorten over time as part of the normal aging process, getting slightly clipped during each cell division until eventually they become so short the cells die or become senescent. This leads to the diminished function of tissues and organs associated with aging. It makes sense, then, that older people have shorter telomeres.

People living with chronic stress, who tend to age rapidly during the period of stress (picture how quickly U.S. presidents go gray once they're in office), also have shorter telomeres.

Researcher Eli Puterman, PhD, psychologist at the University of California San Francisco, found that exercise can maintain telomere length in seriously stressed individuals. He led a study of 62 women past menopause, many of whom were caring for chronically ill spouses or parents. Those who did not exercise had diminished telomere length that correlated to their level of stress. Those who did exercise had longer telomeres and showed no relationship between stress and telomere length.

Exercise Boosts Your Immune System

Dr. David Nieman of Appalachian State University has shown that putting adults of any age into an exercise program led to an immediate and, in some cases, significant reduction in the number of days the test subjects were sick with a cold. This effect was especially pronounced in the elderly, who tend to have reduced immune function anyway, making them more susceptible to a wide variety of common viruses.

> "Putting adults of any age into an exercise program led to an immediate and, in some cases, significant reduction in the number of days the test subjects were sick with a cold."

When you go for a brisk walk, "immune cells come out of the bone marrow, the lungs, and spleen and circulate through the body at a higher rate than normal," Nieman explains. During that period, and for about 3 hours afterward, your body is better at attacking viruses.

For anyone, at any age, the increased immunity and fewer sick days that result from exercise is a "near immediate benefit" of getting off the couch, Dr. Nieman says.

Exercise Reduces Oxidative Stress

There's a paradox here, because exercise has long been known to *increase* oxidative stress. When exercising strenuously, the increased oxygen and energy demands cause the mitochondria to churn out more free radicals, which in turn causes more oxidative damage to your cells. This is especially true for people who exercise strenuously very suddenly—the weekend warrior—who then pay the price in exhaustion, sore muscles, and stiffness. All are signs of acute oxidative stress.

But people who exercise regularly build up an immunity, of sorts, to that oxidative stress, much the way a vaccine might work. The more you experience this kind of exercise-induced free-radical production and resulting oxidative stress, the more your body ramps up production of antioxidant enzymes to gobble up all those free radicals. As a result, consistent exercisers have more antioxidants circulating in their bodies at all times, which means their bodies more effectively squelch oxidative stress of all kinds.

Dr. Nieman recorded this in a survey of 1,000 people age 18 to 85, who were categorized by exercise level and markers of oxidative stress in the blood. Those with the highest exercise levels had "significantly lower" markers of oxidative stress in their blood. These individuals also showed the lowest levels of inflammation, based on protein markers in the blood indicating the presence of inflammation.

Exercise Boosts Your Metabolism
Even the immediate benefits of exercise are longer-lasting than previously thought.

Any time you exercise, your metabolism runs faster while you're actually exerting yourself, causing you to burn more energy. This is part of what makes exercise such a critical part of any weight-loss strategy (besides the important goal of maintaining muscle mass). But a study published in 2011 in *Medicine and Science in Sports and Exercise,* the scientific journal of the American College of Sports Medicine, showed that this engine-revving effect can last a very long time.

In the experiment, male test subjects age 22 to 33 were brought into a lab to live for 24 hours in tightly controlled conditions in a metabolic chamber—a small room that allowed researchers to measure each subject's total caloric intake and energy expenditure while in the room. One 24-hour period was restful and measurements were recorded. Another 24-hour period had all the same variables but included 45 minutes of vigorous exercise. This one bout of exertion "resulted in a significant elevation in postexercise energy expenditure that persisted for 14 hours," the study explained.

In the 14 hours after exercising, the subjects burned an additional 160 calories they wouldn't have burned if they hadn't exercised, the researchers found, increasing the total number of calories expended from exercising by 37 percent.

Exercise Increases Brain Size

Kirk Erickson, PhD, psychologist and aging researcher at the University of Pittsburgh, has conducted several studies showing that exercise has a direct impact on the size of the brain.

In one study, published in 2011 in the *Proceedings of the National Academy of Sciences,* Dr. Erickson divided a group of 120 adults age 55 to 80 into two equal groups. One group spent a year doing stretching and toning exercises three times a week, and the other did 40 minutes of moderate-intensity walking 3 days a week for a year.

At the end of the study, people in the group who had walked three times a week showed a 2 percent increase in the volume of the hippocampus, the region of the brain that converts short-term memory into long-term memories. This is also the first area of the brain to deteriorate in Alzheimer's disease. The group that did not walk, on the other hand, experienced a 1.4 percent decline in the volume of the hippocampus—the typical annual loss in volume of the hippocampus in people who don't exercise. Increases in hippocampal size are tied to improved memory and other measurements of cognitive function.

> "People ... who had walked three times a week showed a 2 percent increase in the volume of the hippocampus."

In another study published in 2008 by Dr. Ross Andel, PhD in gerontology and associate professor at the School of Aging Studies at the University of South Florida, found that regular exercise in midlife cut the risk of developing dementia three decades later by up to 66 percent.

How much is enough? Even walking a mile a day can protect the brain's function later in life, studies show. And the benefits also begin to accrue almost immediately. In an article published in the *Journal of the American Society on Aging* in 2011, Dr. Erickson and Andrea M. Weinstein, a graduate student in his lab, wrote that "a mere six months of regular walking is sufficient to show enhanced brain volume and function."

Exercise Enhances Your Sleep

A review of published studies on the subject of sleep and exercise, published in 2010 in the *American Journal of Lifestyle Medicine,* concluded that aerobic and resistance exercise at levels that meet national recommendations improve a person's quality of sleep. And doing even more exercise, the authors say, appears to improve sleep even further.

This can offer a lot of relief to many people. It's very common for sleep patterns to change as people age and for sleep to be less restful and more disrupted. Yet sleep is critical for physical, mental, and emotional health, and chronic lack of sleep can play a role in aging. Good-quality sleep, on the other hand, has a compound effect on a patient's health and well-being.

A study published in 2010 in the journal *Sleep Medicine,* which was led by Dr. Kathryn J. Reid, neurologist at Northwestern University with a research interest in sleep, found that even people with chronic insomnia could markedly improve their sleep quality and duration by exercising. In the experiment, 10 women age 55 and older went through a 16-week exercise program, beginning with 6 weeks of conditioning exercise sessions to build up their stamina, followed by 10 weeks of 30- to 40-minute workouts 3 or 4 times a week. The subjects exercised at 75 percent of their maximum heart rate, either walking, riding a stationary bicycle, or using a treadmill, in what was described as "moderate-intensity" aerobic physical activity. The exercise participants, as well as seven subjects in a control group who did not exercise, were also given counseling in effective sleep habits and behaviors.

After 16 weeks, compared with the control group of nonexercisers, the subjects who engaged in the exercise program were sleeping an average of 1¹/₄ hours longer each night. They also had improved sleep continuity, fewer depressive symptoms (which often accompany both age and lack of sleep), and reported a better quality of life.

The idea that you can achieve better sleep, a better mood, and a better life in just 16 weeks, just by exercising, is pretty remarkable.

Part of what I like about Dr. Reid's sleep study is how slowly the participants ramped up their exercise regime: they started with just 5 to 10 minutes of exercise 3 or 4 times a week at just 55 percent of their peak heart rate, which is a pretty light workout just about anyone could manage. They did a bit more each week, so that by the end of the conditioning period 6 weeks later, most of the participants were completing moderate-intensity workouts for 40 minutes 3 or 4 times a week—and did that for 10 more weeks. That's fantastic.

Many people would struggle to increase their level of exercise that consistently without the pressure of logs to fill out and researchers following their efforts. But this kind of slow increase in exercise duration is the right approach, even if it's a little faster than many people could achieve on their own. Exercise and behavior scientists say the biggest problem for most people when it comes to exercising is that they don't start slowly enough, so sticking with an exercise program becomes difficult. The next two chapters help you understand more about the process of initiating an exercise regime and doing it in a way that will help you stick with it—for life.

Exercise Helps Regulate Appetite

There's a host of research about the role exercise plays in appetite control and stimulation. Unfortunately, not all of that data is consistent. For example, studies have shown that after exercising, some people get the urge to eat, and the calories they ingest more than make up for the calories they burn during the exercise.

But other people appear to have the opposite reaction: exercise reduces their interest in food. In numerous studies, intense aerobic activity, especially for 60 minutes or longer, has been shown to reduce a person's appetite. This is because blood is diverted away from the digestive system to other parts of the body that need it. But levels of a key appetite-stimulating hormone also decrease, so less of it reaches the brain. Usually within an hour, though, hunger returns. And sometimes with a vengeance.

So how is this helpful? Because physical activity makes your hunger and appetite systems more sensitive and responsive, possibly by affecting neurons in the brain.

Dr. Neil King, professor at Queensland University of Technology in Brisbane, Australia, has done extensive research on the role of exercise in appetite control and weight management. In a study he published in 2010 in the *American Journal of Clinical Nutrition,* Dr. King noted that exercise made food cues—both hunger and satiety—more pronounced.

During the study, he wrote, "The participants had a higher [before breakfast] hunger level at the end of the 12-week period, yet a breakfast meal of identical nutritional composition caused a greater immediate reduction in this hunger and maintained the level of suppression." In other words, subjects who exercised felt hungrier, but food was more satisfying and filling. Over time, some appetite experts believe, having more clear sensations of hunger and satiety can help people regulate their food intake better by more clearly defining the body's signals for when to eat and when to stop.

Calories Burned and Consumed

Don't guess how many calories you've burned, look it up! Lots of free apps and online calculators are available. Check out healthstatus.com/calculate/cbc.

The hard part is to not overeat after exercise. Dr. Eric Doucet with the University of Ottawa, who holds a PhD in physiology and endocrinology, found that people dramatically overestimate the number of calories they burn during exercise. In a study published in 2010 in the *Journal of Sports Medicine and Physical Fitness,* test subjects estimated they'd used three or four times the number of calories they actually had. Calculated another way, when test subjects were asked to consume the amount of food they thought would equal the number of calories they had expended during exercise, they ate two or three times too much!

The following table shows how many calories are burned after
20 minutes of some common exercises for a 150-pound person,
compared with the calories found in some familiar snacks.

Exercise	Calories	Food	Calories
Elliptical trainer	258	Blueberry muffin (Sam's Club)	540
Stationary bike, vigorous	258	Large soft pretzel	483
Running, 6 mph	228	Trail mix with chocolate chips, $1/_2$ cup	353
Zumba	180	Starbucks grande Frappuccino, no whip	240
Jogging	159	Almond granola bar	140
Aerobics, low impact	138	Orange juice, chilled, 8 ounces	110
Tennis, singles	138	Medium (7- or 8-inch) banana	104
Yoga (Ashtanga)	117	Cottage cheese, 2%, $1/_2$ cup	101
Walking, 3 mph	99	Large hard-boiled egg	77

Source: healthstatus.com/calculate/cbc

Always Worth It

The variation in how people's appetites respond to exercise means
some people lose more weight by exercising than others. But the
science is clear that even without weight loss, exercise makes
important contributions to health because of all the other pathways it
stimulates, in the muscles, the cardiovascular system, and the brain,
among others.

The important message is that exercise has multiple benefits, whether or not you notice it, and almost no matter how much you do. When you reach just 10 minutes a day, you're helping yourself age better. If you can build up to doing that three times a day, even better.

But even if all you can do when you first get going is 5 brisk minutes on the stationary bike between household tasks and child-wrangling, you're establishing the habit, and that's what matters. Don't be put off by programs suggesting you have to do more than that to make a difference. It's true, you'll get more of a benefit—more time on the clock—if you can reach federal guideline levels, but don't worry if you have to take your time to get there.

If you let yourself build up slowly, rather than aiming for a washboard stomach next month, you'll naturally and easily get to a point where you're exercising, at least in part, because it makes you feel good. And *that* will make you keep doing it.

> "But even if all you can do when you first get going is 5 brisk minutes on the stationary bike between household tasks and child-wrangling, you're establishing the habit, and that's what matters."

Moderation Mix

Reading about the many positive effects of exercise on aging well is one thing, but what can you do if you spend your days sitting at a desk, don't belong to a gym, and have no sidewalks in your community? How can you start exercising in a way that keeps you engaged and motivated so you can benefit for the rest of your life?

The first thing you need to know is how much exercise it takes to actually make a difference. Federal guidelines suggest two ideal scenarios each week: 150 minutes of moderate-intensity exercise plus strength and resistance exercises, such as sit-ups, push-ups, or light free weights, or 75 minutes of vigorous physical activity plus strength and resistance exercises. Because 92 percent of the population isn't doing that, it doesn't seem like a particularly reasonable goal to start with.

But does doing less make a difference? Absolutely. Federal guidelines, which are formulated with a great deal of input from scientists, exist to give a formula for what's optimal, what your goal should be. But that doesn't mean doing less than the guidelines is meaningless.

Aging experts agree that doing anything is better than nothing. Almost no matter what you do, it will make a difference as long as you stick with it. You can take your time to work your way up to a more vigorous exercise plan, as long as you do it in a way that keeps you going and doesn't feel like a burden. Part of the problem with establishing an exercise program is that it's often the first thing you give up when life gets complicated—and life will always get complicated. Yet that's when you need exercise the most.

I watched my husband start his current exercise routine in—no kidding—5-minute increments 10 years ago. So I know ordinary people, even those who think they don't have time to exercise or have never been able to stick with an exercise program before, can easily establish this lifelong—and life-lengthening—habit. They just have to take the right approach.

The science suggests that exercise should start with the goal of aging well, not trying to get a beach-buff body by summer. Building a foundation of fitness, at the cellular level, keeps you strong and youthful for decades to come. And you may, in the end, still end up with that killer beach body you want.

But to start, *exercising doesn't have to be painful*. It just has to be consistent and long term, like brushing your teeth, taking blood pressure medication, or anything else you do religiously because you know it will yield benefits in the future. Exercise needs to be one of those things.

As the previous chapter showed, the science supports this idea: as soon as you start walking around the block, immune cells rush into your bloodstream and start to protect you from illness. When you start to sweat, levels of natural antioxidants start rising in your body. And just a little bit of walking every day can protect your brain from shrinking, your telomeres from shortening, and your arteries from hardening.

The exercise that will improve your health, slow your aging, and lengthen your life isn't difficult—and it shouldn't hurt. In fact, it should feel good, and it *can* feel good. After all, humans were designed to be active; it's our default setting. Getting there is what matters, and for that, you can take your time to get it right.

You may think you need to join a gym and sweat on an exercise bike for 40 minutes every other day to have an impact on your health, but that's not the case. It's not that exercising at this level would be bad for you—quite the contrary—but it's more than many people can sustain indefinitely. Plus, in terms of aging well, the majority of the benefit of exercise comes at a much lower level.

The Baltimore Longitudinal Study on Aging (BLSA) is about as clear as a piece of science can get when it comes to exercise. As an epidemiological study, the BLSA doesn't look for answers inside cells or tissues, but rather looks at patterns of behavior and outcomes across a population to draw a conclusion. It's sort of like the "Ask the Audience" lifeline on *Who Wants to Be a Millionaire*. Your guidance comes from the general pattern of many rather than specific answers from just one.

In the case of exercise, the BLSA clearly shows that moderate physical activity—even less than what you might think—is where the biggest benefit lies.

"When people talk about physical activity, they always think about jogging or, you know, doing intense physical activity," explains National Institute on Aging's Luigi Ferrucci. "The real difference—the *huge* difference—is between the couch potato and those who walk .... Because ten minutes of walking is hugely different in terms of [aging] risk compared to staying home and watching television."

> "'The real difference—the *huge* difference—is between the couch potato and those who walk [ten minutes a day].'"

Moderate exercise can, quite simply, help you live longer. In late 2012, researchers from Brigham and Women's Hospital in Boston published an analysis of a group of National Cancer Institute studies that had followed more than 650,000 people from age 21 to 90 over many years. They divided up the subjects based on exercise level per week, and compared that data to recorded deaths. They found that walking just 75 minutes a week (about 11 minutes a day!) was associated with living nearly two years longer than people who didn't walk at all. Walking 150 minutes a week (about 21 minutes a day) for normal-weight individuals was associated with living 7.2 years longer. Lifespan benefits were seen across all levels of BMI.

Dr. Neiman's research shows that the biggest benefit comes when people reach the level of walking briskly 30 minutes a day. But that 30 minutes can be broken into 10-minute increments and still accumulate the same benefits. So taking a 10-minute walk in the morning, just in your street clothes, another one at lunch, and another after work is good enough to be highly protective as you age—and a totally realistic goal to pursue. Neiman likes to quote the renowned fitness expert Dr. Kenneth Cooper, who famously said, "Walk your dog every day, even if you don't have one."

If you can start walking every day—or just doing 10 minutes on the stationary bike or treadmill once or twice a day—it may not feel like you're doing anything beneficial. And it may not get you into a bikini. But if you're consistent, it *will* help keep you out of a nursing home.

To start off, you need to find the level of exertion your body is dialed to right now, and do that. If you begin with a manageable goal and stick with it, you can increase the amount of exercise you do over time when you feel like it and when it feels good to ramp up a bit. Every time you do a little more, you're pushing that nursing home farther down the pike.

Cumulative Crunches

It's a good thing aging comes with a long time frame. *The Biggest Loser,* with a weigh-in every week? Forget it. What we should all be aiming for is to be the biggest winner two, three, or four decades from now, which means you can take your time getting there. You have the luxury of starting small and building up your physical strength and endurance over time.

Just like compound interest on a credit card, there is a cumulative effect to the small steps you take throughout your life aimed at aging well, especially when it comes to exercise. In a study published in 2011 in the *American Journal of Preventive Medicine,* a trio of PhDs from England and Australia assessed "whether the beneficial effects of physical activity accumulate over life." They looked at data on 2,400 men and women from the UK Medical Research Council National Survey of Health and Development. All the subjects had been born in March 1946 and were evaluated intermittently throughout their life.

In addition to the many bits of data that had been gathered about this group over the decades, the authors found that various exercises and strength tests had also been performed on the subjects at ages

36, 43, and 53. And all had been asked a variety of questions about their exercise habits. The study put these two pieces of data together to determine the effect of exercise habits at ages 36 and 43 and on strength and fitness at age 53. The participants in the study were just normal people the researchers classified into three groups of the least, moderately, and most active, based on their participation in leisure activities, exercise, and sports.

The last fitness tests had been done in 1999, but none of them had been used for any research or to draw any conclusions. The authors of the journal article began evaluating this data in 2010 and described the evidence as "robust." Even after adjusting for gender, weight, education level, and health problems, they found the benefits of physical activity were cumulative across adulthood.

"Increased activity should be promoted early in adulthood to ensure the maintenance of physical performance in later life," the authors wrote.

In his book, *The Compound Effect, SUCCESS Magazine* publisher Darren Hardy extols the cumulative approach to every aspect of life. Hardy is right on the money with his advice to do small things, one by one, and let them work for you over time: "even though the results are massive, the steps, in the moment, don't feel significant ... they're almost imperceptible."

The only problem with this advice is that people have a hard time starting small because small steps often don't show measurable results right away. But that's not the way to think of it. Rather than focus on the results of your exercise, think of it as maintenance work. Taking small steps toward healthy aging is like putting oil in your car or keeping your kitchen tidy. Aging needs the same attention: if you don't keep up, the result isn't pretty.

> "Aging needs the same attention: if you don't keep up, the result isn't pretty."

Caring for yourself in a way that will improve your future years, and make you look younger and feel better than you otherwise would, does not need to feel overwhelming. Instead, if you make a conscious effort to think about your life as a one-way race from here to there, you can make a conscious decision to slow down in the beginning of the race to save yourself for the home stretch.

It's really the fundamental concept of prevention, but in today's instant-result, pleasure-only world, even a concept as basic as that has come to seem like a daunting challenge that can only make your life today less enjoyable. But not if you figure out a prevention plan uniquely tailored to fit you and your lifestyle.

Now that you know how complex aging is, and how the process of aging begins with tiny cellular changes, you understand that the way you'll feel in the future will be magnified by what you do earlier in life, good or bad. Because the processes that contribute to aging are so interrelated, ignoring one aspect of your health or well-being invariably influences another. Each choice sets in motion not just one factor in the aging process, but many.

So if you overeat, for example, you not only get the effect of excess fat, which can lead to diabetes, you also get the effect of increased oxidative stress, which leads to mitochondrial decay, which leads to greater cell senescence, which leads to tissue damage and a greater risk of cancer.

But the reverse is also true: if you *improve* one aspect of your health consistently over time, you positively influence multiple aging factors. If you exercise consistently, for example, building up slowly and sticking with it over many years, your body will produce more of its own antioxidants, which will decrease the amount of damage to your cells from oxidative stress, leading to better tissue and organ function, and a reduced risk of cancer. It's processes like this that make exercise so critical to keeping you healthy later in life.

The other important point about the cumulative benefits of exercise is that, as Dr. Nieman pointed out, the people who do it consistently tend to *like* doing it, and that keeps them going. It may take a few weeks to get that "I like this" feeling, but it will come. You don't need to become an exercise freak to feel that way, either. You just need to be smart about building up *gradually*.

First Steps

Remember the warning about the weekend warrior, who goes out on the weekend and overdoes it, stimulating a cascade of oxidative stress–induced injury and discomfort? Whatever you do, *don't do that*. Don't do more than you can handle or more than what feels manageable. Better yet, stop even before you feel like you've had enough, when you feel like you could keep exercising. That will minimize the damage caused by oxidative stress, which will keep you from feeling spent or in pain. That will dramatically increase the chances you'll want to exercise again!

So if all you can handle is a 10-minute walk three times a week, commit to do that and feel proud you're doing something to benefit your future self. Don't feel embarrassed or inadequate when a Spandex-clad, sweat-drenched hottie goes running by you. For all you know, he or she also started with just 10 minutes of exercise 3 days a week. The key thing is picking whatever level of exercise you know you can do over and over.

Even doing a little bit will make you feel good, and your enthusiasm for taking care of yourself will grow—as Jim's has, exponentially, in the past few years. Once you start to enjoy your walks (or whatever exercise you chose to do) in this way, you'll want to do even more so you can keep that feeling of accomplishment and pride. That's human nature. Eventually your new habit will become an urge, and that's when you should add a little bit more time to your routine— do another lap around the block or add a few crunches and curls when you get home. Whatever it is, however insignificant it may seem to you at the time, it's anything but insignificant because you're sticking with it and moving forward.

> "Don't feel embarrassed or inadequate when some Spandex-clad, sweat-drenched hottie goes running by you. For all you know, he or she also started with just 10 minutes of exercise 3 days a week."

It's Never Too Late

If cumulative exercise is the key to prevention, what do you do if you're already past midlife, or you're already experiencing age-related health problems? Well, you start by not worrying that you're past the point of no return. Even bed-ridden nursing home residents have shown dramatic improvement from doing moderate exercise. Studies have shown that exercise means spending less time in bed, showing more alertness, having a better outlook, and more.

"It's never too late to start," says Dr. Mark Tarnopolsky, of McMaster University in Ontario. He is one of many experts who expressed this opinion.

Aging is always happening, from roughly puberty all the way through the day you die. Anytime you intervene along that continuum, you slow the aging process from that point onward. So if you're 65 and just starting to realize you want to do something to improve the quality, if not the length, of the rest of your life, you still have years to get it right. Maybe not as many years, but you can make a significant difference.

This is what happened in the study done by Simon Melov at the Buck Institute: the average age of the older adults who enrolled in the study's exercise program was 70, and after 6 months, they had improved their muscle strength by 50 percent. They also had nearly totally reversed, in their cells, the age-related genetic markers for muscle loss.

Prevention, of course, is always the ideal, because it's easier to stay healthy than to get sick and try to fix it. The problem with that rule is it stems from the benefit of hindsight: you don't know that prevention is easier until you actually get sick, or weak, or overweight and then have a really hard time reversing it. That's when it seems like it sure would've been easier to walk 10 minutes a day or eat more fruit.

But the benefits of exercise remain multifactorial even later in life. It's not just your muscles that get stronger.

Researchers at the Mayo Clinic, for example, evaluated the exercise patterns and development of mild cognitive impairment, or early dementia, in 1,324 older adults, age 70 to 89, as part of an ongoing population-based study. Their results, published in 2010 in the journal *Archives of Neurology,* showed that "any frequency of moderate intensity exercise carried out in either midlife or late life was associated with a reduced [risk] of mild cognitive impairment."

But perhaps nothing makes it clearer that it's never too late to exercise than the plethora of studies showing the impact exercise has on the survival of cancer patients. A large review of published papers on cancer patients conducted from 1950 through August 2011 was recently published in the *Journal of the National Cancer Institute.* These were all observational studies, not clinical trials. Some were very specific in their focus on a particular kind of cancer and, therefore, evaluated only a small group of patients. But the authors of the 2012 review found that of the 45 articles published on the impact of exercise on cancer patients, 27 showed a link between exercise and reduced mortality.

That moderate exercise could have such a big impact in such a dire situation shows the incredible power you have to change your future, especially if you're healthy, because you have all the tools at your disposal to work on keeping it that way. I have personally observed, in the past decade, just how rewarding that effort can be.

How Jim Did It

I didn't realize it at the time, but the science of exercise has played out in my house. So has the psychology of exercise.

Through the first half of our 21-year marriage, it seemed like Jim and I were never on the same exercise schedule. I'd go through bouts of exercising extensively for a period of time, while he was being more or less inactive. I remember his commenting at the time that he admired me for working out so diligently and wished he could exercise the way I did. But then there were times when he would get on an exercise kick and I would be the rhymes-with-*hazy* one—studiously avoiding being around when he was working out so I wouldn't feel so guilty. We exercised in relation to whatever life had in store: when our jobs got busy, or other commitments took over, exercise fell by the wayside.

We never worked out together, and neither of us found a program that stuck. Jim's default was doing some version of the rowing machine, the exercise bike, and exercises or weights, while I floundered between our makeshift basement gym, swimming, running, and even boot camp. After our first daughter was born in 1998, we both pretty much stopped exercising. We felt terrible—but doesn't everyone when they have a baby?

Then about 10 years ago, Jim started exercising in a way that seemed, to me, sort of ridiculous. We had a toddler and a new baby and—you guessed it—no time. But he would come home from work and say, "You know, I'm just going to go downstairs and do ten minutes on the bike because I think I need it. But I'll be right back up to help."

And, uh, what good does that do when you could be helping me put the kids to bed? is what I would think to myself, in the way wives do. But what would come out, instead, was, "Okay, Honey." All I wanted was for him to come back up and help me change some diapers. Forget this exercise folly.

> "I'm just going to go downstairs and do ten minutes on the bike because I think I need it."

But darned if he didn't keep doing it, three times a week, week in and week out. It really was just 10 minutes at first—he'd barely break a sweat. But he'd come upstairs all proud of himself for "working out." Frankly, it was pretty hilarious, in the way wives find their husbands hilarious.

"That's great, Honey," I'd say. "Here's the baby."

But then his 10 minutes turned to 15, with 12 minutes on the bike or rowing machine and some sit-ups, too. Then, a year later, his 15 minutes turned to 20 minutes, with some push-ups added in. And by that time, he was coming upstairs pretty sweaty. But the baby (then our third) didn't care, so I handed him over.

Around the time the fog of babyhood began to lift, and our lives were returning to some version of normal, I began to notice, with some amazement, that Jim was always in a better mood, he had more energy, and he was more patient with the kids. (Of course I said none of this to him.) The days that really got my attention were the ones when he would come home at 8, after an 11-hour day of crisis and deadlines, looking exhausted, kiss the kids, and then say, "I'm going downstairs to exercise. I feel awful, but I'll feel worse if I don't."

I'm not going to lie and say I didn't sometimes resent that 20 minutes he took for himself. *HEY! Where's MY 20 minutes?*

But I came to realize that Jim had carved out those 20 minutes the only time of the day he could, and if it happened to be when three kids were melting down, well, there's wasn't anything he could do about that. And the fact that he was so helpful when he came back upstairs made all the difference—more helpful, and happier about it, too. There can't be a wife on the planet who doesn't appreciate that.

I eventually decided I need to find my own 20 minutes, usually early in the morning because unlike Jim, I don't mind getting up and going right away, and it was the only time I could steal. But I still haven't learned to build up slowly. When I exercise I tend to do 20 or 30 minutes right off the bat and stick with it for a while. But I can't sustain it.

I am learning from watching my husband, however, who nearly a decade later, still diligently exercises three or four times a week, but his workouts have grown to be about 45 minutes—shorter if he doesn't have the time and longer if he can swing it. He has a host of improvements to show for it: he feels stronger, looks younger, sleeps better (better than me, too), is less stressed, and never gets a cold, even with little kids in the house.

I bet his telomeres are longer, too.

Jim's Workout Routine

Jim's workout consists of 15 to 18 minutes on the stationary bike, a 2-minute break, 10 to 15 minutes on the rowing machine (he uses a Concept2), 5 minutes of sit-ups and push-ups, and 10 to 15 minutes of free weights.

After the past few years watching this transformation, I have developed a longer-term outlook on my physical fitness. I do not beat myself up when I don't exercise; I always make an effort to do it, but my approach is to do whatever I can whenever I can. I'll take the 25-minute walk to work on a nice day rather than catching a ride with Jim, for example. Or if 10 minutes are all I have, I'll get on the bike for 10 minutes.

I'm not as consistent as Jim is, but I'm more active than I was, and I'm getting there. I'm only 2 years into it; I've got time.

Part 4

Boost Your Brain

One-Track Mind

It's understandable that people often think about their brain as aging separately from their body. It often *seems* like two different processes.

Getting older usually means getting a little slower, weaker, and heavier; showing a few wrinkles; going gray; and perhaps, if you're unlucky, developing such debilities as diabetes, arthritis, hearing or vision loss, heart disease, digestive problems, or cancer. On the other hand, a whole different set of issues affect the brain later in life, such as memory problems, dementia, Alzheimer's disease, Parkinson's, or other neurological disorders.

The symptoms of body aging and brain aging appear to develop on parallel tracks, independently, and not necessarily at the same time. You can develop dementia even when your body is fine physically, and your body can deteriorate even as your brain stays fully functional and engaged.

But the latest science is squarely focused on the powerful connection between aging of the body and brain, not only as people approach their upper age brackets but also throughout life. How well you care for, listen to, and respond to your body in your 40s, 50s, and 60s is closely associated with how well your brain will function in your final years or decades—and vice versa.

Body and brain are, in fact, on the same track, responding to the same healthy habits and bad behaviors, including these:

- Physical activity
- Nutrition
- Stress

But the brain needs extra help, too. It's also affected by how you actually use your brain when you're young—what you think, how you feel, and how much you learn. Studies show that cognitive health in later years is also influenced by the following:

- Continual intellectual engagement
- Having a sense of purpose in life
- Staying in contact with close friends
- Conscientiousness
- Spirituality

To keep your brain from deserting you before the party's over, you have to take care of your body *and* your brain. Both can be done, and doing both makes a difference no matter when you start or how incrementally you dive in. But like any savings account, the earlier you get going, the more power you have to put time back on your clock.

You don't see yourself aging when you look in the mirror one week to the next, but you know you *are* aging ever so slowly, even imperceptibly. It's only once in a while that you look at yourself and realize you don't look—or feel, or think—like you used to. Likewise, when you take small steps to slow down that process, to boost your brain and support your cells, you probably won't notice the change week to week, but over time, they add up to make a real difference. That's when you look in the mirror and think, *You know, I look pretty good, and I feel pretty good, too.*

> "To keep your brain from deserting you before the party's over, you have to take care of your body *and* your brain."

Reserve Army

The science of brain aging has made incredible advances, thanks to imaging technology, which can take detailed pictures of structures in the brain and even which parts of the brain are most active when you're using it. This has been especially valuable for comparing brain function at different ages. When an older person is asked to do a calculation, for example, a larger portion of the brain lights up than when a younger person performs the same task. The older brain is less efficient, but it compensates by calling on other parts of the brain to step in and help.

It's a little like lifting an arm chair to move it across the room: a younger person can do it alone using his or her own strength, but an older person needs someone else to help lift the chair and move it.

But brain scans can be maddening, too: they show how much we still don't know about why and how some people develop memory problems, dementia, and diseases like Alzheimer's. In theory, if you look at the brain of a cognitively diminished person (the scientific term is *demented*), it should look different from the brain of a normally functioning individual. The demented brain might be smaller, have sections of dead tissue or holes where brain tissue has dissolved, contain abnormal protein clumps, or some combination of these. But it turns out that the way a brain looks on a scan may not bear any relationship to how functional the owner of that brain really is.

My own father is a good example. He was a brilliant historian, intellectually curious and active, but also deeply engaged in many aspects of culture and life. A year before he died at age 89, I took him to have a brain scan because of severe mobility issues and exhaustion he had developed quite suddenly. The radiologist remarked to my father's internist that his brain scan looked like that of his own father—who was in the advanced stages of Alzheimer's disease. Yet there was my father, a little slow and sleepy at times, but otherwise chatting, joking, sharp, and clearly enjoying life. Outwardly, he seemed to be aging pretty well. But his brain scan was far from ideal.

"You can have two brains, and they both have lots of Alzheimer's pathology, but you see that one person was severely demented during life and the other one had no symptoms," said Dr. William Jagust, neuroscientist at the University of California, Berkeley. "The question is, how can this be?"

The emerging answer is that the brain has something called *cognitive reserve*. Essentially, this is the brain's ability to keep functioning despite deterioration. Cognitive reserve is like the brain's built-in backup system. It allows the parts of the brain that aren't damaged to take over for the parts that are. To understand how that happens, it helps to know a little bit about the biology of the human brain.

"Outwardly, he seemed to be aging pretty well. But his brain scan was far from ideal."

It may weigh only 3 pounds, but a person can have a hundred billion nerves cells, called neurons, in the brain, and a quadrillion points of connection among those cells. It's those connections, like a computer motherboard, that power all your thinking, analyzing, dreaming, remembering, smelling, seeing, moving, and breathing.

Neurons are specialized cells that look kind of like trees: one end holds a bunch of branches like the crown of a tree. The middle section is like a long, thin trunk. And the far end has more branching but is less dense—more like the roots of a tree. Neurons communicate by sending tiny, electrically charged molecules across gaps (or synapses), where the branches of one tree (called dendrites) meet the roots (or axons) of the next tree. These electrochemical signals power your life.

Some people have more nerve endings in their brains than other people. They may have more neurons—essentially a thicker forest with more trees—or they may have especially dense, complex branching at the ends of each nerve, like the top of a big, healthy shade tree.

But some people have fewer neurons and a looser structure of nerve endings, like a tree that lets lots of sunshine through. With fewer neurons and nerve endings, the brain has fewer overall connections.

These structural differences are at the heart of cognitive reserve and help explain why some people's brains are more or less vulnerable to cognitive decline. As we age, the branches of nerve endings in our brains gradually get pruned back—by disease, by injury, or simply by lack of use. It happens to everyone.

But if you have a lot of connections to begin with, you'll have more connections left, even after years of pruning. This is how Dr. Paul Nussbaum, clinical neuropsychologist at the University of Pittsburgh Medical School, explains it: "If you think of Alzheimer's as a weed whacker, it's going to take a whole heck of a lot longer to get through a jungle than through a few palm trees." Those remaining undamaged parts of the brain are your cognitive reserve, and they can pick up the slack for the parts that *are* damaged.

The brain does not just accept all the age-related deterioration it experiences without fighting back. It has various defense mechanisms, such as proteins that generate neuron growth in response to certain behaviors like exercise. But the most common defense against cognitive decline is that the brain figures out a workaround.

> "The brain does not just accept all the age-related deterioration it experiences without fighting back."

If a young, healthy person's brain sends a signal directly from point A to point B, for example, an older person might have to make that same communication by sending a signal first from A to C and *then* from C to B. That's why more of the brain lights up in the MRI of an older person performing a thinking task.

"They are bringing different parts of their brain online," Jagust explains.

It may be a sign of inefficiency and age, but when a bigger portion of an older brain lights up when performing a task, it's also a great sign of resilience. The more healthy neurons a person's brain can call on to perform a workaround, answer a question, or recall a memory, the longer that person will be able to function independently and enjoy life.

If everyone has at least some deterioration in their brains as they age, then everyone needs plenty of cognitive reserve.

So how do you get it?

The biggest factor influencing cognitive reserve may be one that you can't do a whole lot about at this point: a higher level of education. All that time spent learning when you were young actually built brain tissue, one connection at a time. Although much of the brain's growth stops in your 20s, every time you learn something new—and this is true throughout life—that learning stimulates new pathways between neurons to encode and remember that bit of knowledge, that face, or that experience. Learning can even cause the generation of completely new neurons.

This helps explain why someone like my father, highly educated to begin with and extremely intellectually active throughout life, kept much of his cognitive ability until shortly before he died. As kids, my sister and I used to joke that he had a big brain, and that's why hats were often too small for him. We didn't know how right we were!

Consider a study done by researchers in Germany, who used MRI scans to measure the brains of medical students before and after studying for exams. After months of intense studying, the researchers reported in *The Journal of Neuroscience* in 2006, the amount of gray matter in the students' brains had "increased significantly."

Other studies have shown increases in brain size from consistent learning and practice of various tasks, including learning to play an instrument, speak a new language, or even juggle! Chinese researchers published a study in 2011 in the journal *Proceedings of the National Academy of Sciences* showing that changes can be seen in as little as a few hours of intense learning. The researchers used MRI scans to measure the brains of adult subjects before almost 2 hours of learning new color names and found an increase in the volume of gray matter in the left visual cortex of the subjects' brains, which is the area responsible for discerning color vision.

> "After months of intense studying, ... the amount of gray matter in the students' brains had 'increased significantly.'"

The Friendship Factor

As important as learning is, we can't spend all our days in the library, so luckily, other factors also appear to affect cognitive reserve throughout life. Among the most important are having a large network of close friends, physical activity, physical health, cognitive engagement, and a sense of purpose in life. These are some of the main factors observed by neurologist Dr. David Bennett, director of the Alzheimer's Disease Center at Rush University Medical Center in Chicago.

Dr. Bennett heads up two large population-based studies looking at the causes and conditions of dementia and other kinds of cognitive impairment. One involves about a thousand Catholic clergy, nuns and brothers, while the other follows regular individuals from the community, for a total of about 2,700 people. Everyone entered the study at about age 70 or older, and none had dementia at the outset. All participants also agreed to be regularly evaluated for cognitive decline and then donate their brains to science after their death.

Clock-Cheater Tip

It almost doesn't matter what you learn; it will benefit your brain. But even better is discussing what you've learned with someone else. Some great ways to do that include joining a book club, taking a continuing education seminar at the local university or community college, or taking a class with a chatty friend or two so you're not just learning but also socializing as you learn.

So far, hundreds of participants in the two studies have developed Alzheimer's disease, and Bennett's team has performed more than 1,000 autopsies. Not one brain at the time of death (average age, 87) appeared normal, even though many subjects had displayed normal cognitive function when they died. Bennett has sorted through waves of data analyzing various aspects of these people's lives to draw conclusions about what factors influence a person's rate of cognitive decline, such as activity level, personality, physical health, genetics, and life experience.

Some factors seem to make an aging person do worse in general, no matter what or how severe the existing brain problems might be. Depression does that, for example. Other factors seem to make people do better overall, regardless of underlying pathology, such as general happiness. These factors are a little mysterious because they seem to operate independently of anything else going on in the brain, "like a proxy for something we haven't measured, either good or bad," Bennett says.

But what has clearly emerged from Dr. Bennett's research is the strongly positive effect of having a large social network, especially in people with clear evidence of disease in their brains.

"Social networks is where I'll ask you how many people, other than your spouse and children, do you feel comfortable talking to and confiding in. Not Twitter or Facebook friends, but the number of people [who], if you had a problem, you could call and rely on. That's your network," Bennett says. "It's such a simple concept, but it turns out to be remarkably predictive of all kinds of things."

The bigger a person's social network, the more resistant they are to the effects of brain disease, Bennett says. "It somehow changes the way your brain is responding to the pathology," he says.

It's not really clear why, but neuroscientists like Bennett and Jagust believe it makes sense. "If you think about what your brain was developed for, it was developed for social interaction," Jagust says. So from an evolutionary perspective, creating a strong network of friends *should* enhance overall survival.

Exactly what the mechanism is that controls this isn't known, but Dr. Bennett thinks it might be that making friends—and keeping them—is a challenge, and the brain responds to a challenge by activating all kinds of growth systems and protective measures. Education does that, too, since it clearly is a challenge when you work hard to understand and remember facts, ideas, theories, and solutions.

"From an evolutionary perspective, creating a strong network of friends *should* enhance overall survival."

"It's hard to build a large social network—you've got to nurture it, you've got to be able to deal with all kinds of other people," Bennett says. Doing so, it seems, builds a denser, more resilient brain.

Other cognitive factors that protect your brain over time include the following:

Thinking more: Reading, writing, doing puzzles, playing games— anything that makes your brain work harder increases blood flow to it, bringing oxygen and nutrients that help keep existing connections in place.

Being socially active: Not only does this help build your network of friends, but it also exposes your brain to new experiences and ideas, which—you guessed it—builds and preserves connections in your brain.

Finding something meaningful in life: Having a sense of purpose seems to bring together many of these other factors: it gets you out of the house and exposed to new situations, it makes you interact with others, and it improves your outlook, which decreases the negative effects of depression.

Do Brain-Exercise Programs Work?

There's much conflicting evidence about the kinds of brain-athletics programs being sold today as a way to keep your brain young. Certainly, scientific evidence suggests that using your brain and thinking more in any way is good for you. So in that way, these programs are doing some good. But do memory exercises actually improve your memory? That's not so clear. Some scientific studies have shown that doing certain cognitive training exercises only make you better at that cognitive exercise, but there's little "generalization" to the real world, according to neuroscientist Dr. William Jagust at the University of California, Berkeley. On the other hand, some studies show there is some benefit to everyday life. "The jury is still a little out on this," Jagust says. "There's no evidence that it ... protects from Alzheimer's."

Of course, there also can be a strong component of genetics in someone's risk of developing dementia. There are, for example, variants of a particular gene, called APOE e4, that increase a person's risk of developing cognitive impairment. Early onset Alzheimer's disease can run in families, too. Some scientific studies have shown that dietary interventions on such genetically inclined individuals are not effective. On the other hand, those Scandinavian research projects on identical twins suggests that genetic factors can, in fact, be mitigated by a healthier lifestyle.

But for the vast majority of people, it is behavioral, cognitive, and dietary habits that make the big difference—which means positive interventions can really work.

Small changes made over a long period of time can help your brain weather the inevitable changes that come with age—maybe even in people with an unlucky genetic blueprint.

Nourish Your Neurons

How you use your brain throughout your life—to think, learn, and interact with people—is crucial to your brain health. But that's only one of three elements that play a huge role in keeping your brain functioning normally for as long as possible. You also need a healthy diet and physical activity to keep your neurons nourished and your networks nimble.

In earlier chapters, we've looked at plenty of evidence in support of exercise and proper nutrition. Eating well is good for your cells, while eating poorly or too much damages them bit by bit. And exercise helps maintain many functions in your body, from your muscles all the way down to your mitochondria. Both of these factors also have a significant impact on the health of your brain.

There's probably no clearer example of how dramatically food and fitness affect your cognitive health than a major study done with dogs. Studying canine cognition isn't done just because dogs are man's best friend. Dogs perform more complex cognitive strategies than many animals, have sophisticated brain structures, and develop many of the same age-related physical signatures of cognitive decline people do—including memory loss and conditions similar to Alzheimer's disease in humans. They also process nutrients in much the way humans do. That makes them a great proxy for the study of aging in humans.

Dr. Elizabeth Head, neuroscientist at the Sanders-Brown Center on Aging at the University of Kentucky, looks at how diet, exercise, behavioral experiences, and vaccines work on dogs in order to develop a better understanding of how such factors might affect humans. In one especially revealing study, Dr. Head tracked the brain health of about 50 older beagles for 2 years. The dogs ranged in age from 7 to 11, or old enough that some of them were already showing signs of memory problems and brain deterioration. Head divided the dogs into four groups:

- The control group received standard care, with some interaction with other dogs and some access to large indoor running spaces.
- The second group had the same living conditions as the control group but ate a diet fortified with vitamins and antioxidant-rich foods, such as tomatoes, carrots, citrus, and spinach. They got the same number of calories, however, as the control dogs.
- The third group did not get the special diet but got lots of behavioral enrichment: toys, regular walks outside, and socialization with other dogs.
- The last group got *both* the enriched diet and the behavioral enhancement.

Within a couple weeks, the dogs who were fed the diet alone had already started to show improvement in attention and their ability to learn. "We blinked and said, 'that can't be right,'" Head recalls.

But in subsequent weeks, as the dogs were tested further using various kinds of cognitive tests, the improvements not only lasted, they continued. And not just for this subset of dogs. The dogs who got the behavioral enhancements and exercise did even better than the dogs who ate only the special diet.

Most amazing, though, was that the dogs who got *both* the nutrient-rich food and the behavioral enrichments did best of all.

"They were so good after two years of treatment, they looked no different [from how they had in] the beginning," Head says. "We had totally maintained their cognitive function over two years. They should have been going through a rapid phase of aging; we were essentially able to halt that."

The results were revelatory in several ways; most encouraging to the researchers was realizing that the changes in the dogs' behavior and diet interventions protected their brains in different ways. At the end of the study, the brains of the dogs fed the antioxidant diet contained fewer plaques, which are abnormal clumps of proteins that cause Alzheimer's-like symptoms in dogs. The dogs who got more exercise and social enrichment, however, had just as many plaques as the control dogs who had no diet or behavior enhancements—yet they were still in much better shape cognitively than the control dogs. Why? Because the dogs who had been exercised and socially engaged, it turned out, had lost fewer neurons over the course of the study.

> "'They should have been going through a rapid phase of aging; we were essentially able to halt that.'"

That explains why the group of dogs who got both lifestyle improvements benefitted so much more than either group individually. They got the benefit not only of developing fewer brain plaques, but also of keeping more neurons intact, which enhanced their cognitive reserve. In other words, a good diet is good for you. Exercise is good for you. But the two together are greater than the sum of their parts.

This study clearly shows why making an effort to eat more fruits and vegetables, even if you're already physically fit, will benefit you years or decades from now. Or why walking every day will improve how you age, even if you eat the healthiest of diets right now.

"All the things we did with the food, the exercise, everything, is easily done with people," Head explains. "It's these small changes over time, which as they come together, are hitting multiple pathways in your brain and let you really slow down the aging process."

Healthier Humans

Many studies in humans have also targeted the impact of diet and exercise on brain health. For sheer simplicity and clarity of outcome, of course, it's hard to beat Head's dog experiment. But other research provides additional clues about what kinds of foods may help protect your cognitive future.

> ### Clock-Cheater Tip
> If you're middle aged and already feel like your brain isn't working as well for you, it probably isn't—but it *should* be. Don't ignore it: now is the time to start boosting your intake of vitamin-rich foods and taking steps to reduce your stress. And of course, talk to your doctor about it.

The importance of various micronutrients to brain health has been shown in numerous studies, for example. Some B vitamins influence levels of a particular amino acid in the blood associated with a greater risk of developing Alzheimer's disease. Vitamin D, meanwhile, has been identified as playing a role in processing and cementing memories.

This is one of the main messages delivered in the books, talks, and examining room of Dr. Daniel Amen, psychiatrist, author of numerous books on the brain, and head of the Amen clinics. What you eat and how you live your life, he says, has a direct effect on how well your brain looks. Amen's clinics use a type of brain imagery called a SPECT scan, which doesn't show the structure of the brain, but instead shows the brain's activity level. Some of the pictures are pretty alarming, such as those of 30- and 40-year-olds with what looks like clearly diminished brain activity.

But the before and after pictures are enough to make you throw out everything in your pantry. Once someone has gone through an Amen makeover, which involves getting totally immersed in healthy behaviors and high levels of nutrition, the SPECT pictures of his patients' brains look remarkably improved, even after just a couple months. Their brains appear to be working better in every way.

"Alzheimer's disease starts in the brain before people have any symptoms .... That should scare the socks off all of us," Amen says. "At our clinics, ... usually the brains I see look pretty lousy."

In laboratories nationwide, scientists are finding clear evidence tying brain health to diet. A study conducted by researchers at Oregon Health and Science University in Portland, published in 2012 in the journal *Neurology,* showed that elderly subjects with higher levels of vitamins B, C, D, and E in their blood performed better on various cognitive, attention, and executive function tests. Other studies, meanwhile, have implicated low levels of certain vitamins as increasing one's risk of developing dementia. Researchers have linked slight deficiencies in vitamins such as B_{12}, B_6, and folate, as well as vitamin D and the mineral magnesium to sometimes large jumps in the risk of experiencing early cognitive decline.

How do you get more vitamins into your blood? Easy—by eating more plant-based foods, especially fruits and vegetables. A study published in 2010 in the *American Journal of Geriatric Psychiatry* looked at the effect of fruit and vegetable consumption in a population of Swedish twins. The researchers used data on the twins that had been gathered 30 years before about their fruit and vegetable consumption. They then identified and tested as many of the twins as possible and found a clear pattern across the decades: subjects who had eaten more fruits and vegetables in middle age had a measurably lower risk of dementia 30 years later.

Other researchers are looking at the impact of healthy fats on brain health. Researchers at the University of California Los Angeles tested the blood of more than 1,500 elderly study participants, all free of dementia, for the presence of various vitamins, minerals, and omega-3 fatty acids. Then they measured their brains using MRI scans and tested everyone for cognitive function. The study participants with the lowest levels of omega-3 fatty acids in their blood not only had smaller brain volumes, they also generally scored lower on cognitive ability tests, including measurements of visual memory, problem-solving, and multi-tasking.

The results were published in 2012 in the journal *Neurology* and confirmed findings reported earlier, in 2006, by researchers at the USDA's Human Nutrition Research Center on Aging at Tuft's University in Boston. In that study, a good diet was found to have long-term benefits. Nearly 900 subjects free of dementia and ranging in age from 55 to 88 were ranked by the concentration of DHA, an omega-3 fatty acid, in their blood. When tested 9 years later, the participants who had had the highest levels of DHA in their blood at the beginning of the study period had a 47 percent lower risk of dementia than the other participants.

Clock-Cheater Tip

Don't just look for ways to get more healthy fats in your diet, such as omega-3 fatty acids; look for ways to reduce unhealthy fats, too. Researchers at Oregon Health and Science University in Portland tested 104 elderly subjects with an average age of 87 and found that those with higher levels of trans fats in their blood performed worse on cognitive function tests and had smaller brain volume.

More studies are taking place all the time that evaluate the role specific foods can play in protecting against age-related brain deterioration. Here are three recent notable examples, all from 2012:

Berries: A study published in the *Annals of Neurology* analyzed cognitive function and food consumption among 16,000 nurses being studied in an ongoing epidemiological health survey. The research showed that women who regularly ate berries high in flavonoid antioxidants, such as blueberries and strawberries, lived an average of $2^1/_2$ years longer without cognitive impairment than study participants who didn't eat berries.

Walnuts: A Spanish study published in the *Journal of Alzheimer's Disease* showed that people who eat walnuts regularly score better on memory tests and have better overall cognitive function. Walnuts contain antioxidants and omega-3 fatty acids. The same study also found memory-preserving evidence for consumption of olive oil, coffee, and red wine.

Green tea: A Japanese study, published in the *American Journal of Clinical Nutrition,* found that Japanese seniors who drank the most green tea had the lowest prevalence of cognitive disability. Green tea is high in antioxidants.

These studies—and many more like them from the past decade and longer—are exciting to read and offer great guidance for easy ways to incorporate healthier foods into your diet that will make a big difference to your health for years to come. Start sprinkling walnuts on your cereal, have strawberries as a snack, or drink green tea after lunch, for example. But the studies are so varied, it's hard to sum them up in a simple list. Taken together, they illustrate the power of a more nutritious diet in general, especially one with many plant-based foods, much like the diet Dr. Head fed to her study dogs.

Whatever fruits, vegetables, whole grains, or nuts you happen to find convenient and affordable, start eating them when you can. By doing that, you'll be making microscopic changes to your cells that will help your brain stay healthier in the long run. It doesn't matter if you can only do a little bit here or there at first—just get started now. The earlier you start, the more time you have to accumulate the benefits, one strawberry at a time.

> "The earlier you start, the more time you have to accumulate the benefits, one strawberry at a time."

Inflammation Information

Among the changes that positive dietary and exercise habits bring to your brain—and your body—is the suppression of inflammation. Chronic inflammation is a condition identified as a factor in aging and age-related diseases, yet it's not well understood. The science is so new—even unclear—that some aging experts are unwilling to call inflammation a clear-cut risk factor in the aging process. Yet countless other scientists, doctors, and health experts regularly identify it as one.

What is clear is that inflammation appears in aging brains. What's not so clear is the role it plays in developing brain disease and cognitive decline.

When most people think of inflammation, they think of their ankle swelling after twisting it or some other obvious response of the immune system to an injury. Chronic inflammation is more insidious: it's a low-level but near-constant immune system response, at the cellular level, to damage inflicted on cells and tissues by oxidative stress, cell senescence, and cell death.

When poor lifestyle habits cause these kinds of microscopic damage, you can't see it with the naked eye and probably won't even notice it until it builds up enough that you're visibly aging—or you get sick. But don't be fooled; as soon as your less-than-ideal behaviors disrupt your body's carefully balanced environment, damaged cells start releasing signaling proteins called *cytokines* that alert the immune system something is wrong. The immune system mobilizes to repair whatever damage it might find, and the process of repairing or cleaning out that damage causes microscopic inflammation.

Chronically poor lifestyle habits (overeating, for example, or not getting enough vitamins, minerals, and antioxidants) turn this cycle of damage and repair into a constant assault on your cells. This creates a continuous state of low-level inflammation wherever the damage is happening, or possibly throughout the body.

Testing for certain proteins in the blood, such as c-reactive protein, can detect the presence of inflammation. It's a warning sign when c-reactive protein is elevated in your blood because it suggests systemic inflammation, or low-level tissue-swelling somewhere in your body. Over long periods of time, this kind of continued immune response is associated with greater risk of heart disease, cancer, and other conditions of aging.

But here's the problem scientists are struggling with: does inflammation contribute to the development of disease, or is it just another repercussion of an unhealthy choice, such as smoking or eating too much fatty food? Many scientists would say the jury is still out on that. "There's increasing evidence that it's linked to aging, but it's hard to pin down what's going on," says Dr. Brian Kennedy, president of the Buck Institute for Research on Aging.

Either way, it's clear that if you have elevated levels of inflammation, something in your lifestyle isn't right. Cellular damage is happening inside you, somewhere, and you should find a way to slow it down.

This process of inflammation also happens in the brain. The brain doesn't swell from chronic inflammation, but it does get an increased level of cytokines, protein molecules that are a marker for inflammation, explains Donna M. Wilcock, neuroscientist at the Sanders-Brown Center on Aging at the University of Kentucky. Those levels of cytokines are higher in the presence of dementia and Alzheimer's disease, and scientists like Dr. Wilcock are trying to figure out why.

> "If you have elevated levels of inflammation, something in your lifestyle isn't right. Cellular damage is happening inside you, somewhere, and you should find a way to slow it down."

"We think what's happening is there may be a two-hit process going on in Alzheimer's disease, which is that if you have inflammation processes early in your life, from an unhealthy lifestyle, a bad diet, and a lot of chronic inflammation, then you start to develop some of the Alzheimer's pathologies when you're old," she says. In other words, having chronic inflammation when you're young makes you vulnerable to inflammation in the brain when you're older, which appears to play a role in the development of Alzheimer's disease and other types of cognitive impairment that comes with aging.

"If you can change the inflammation that's happening in your body, you're going to change the inflammation in your brain," says Dr. Wilcock. "This is a whole body phenomenon."

Brain Healing

How can you heal your brain? You need to start with an understanding of how the brain works and responds to the signals it gets and the nutrition it's given. Hopefully, this chapter has clarified some of the factors that matter the most.

In a presentation at a 2012 brain health forum sponsored by the American Society on Aging, Dr. Paul D. Nussbaum, clinical neuro-psychologist from the University of Pittsburgh School of Medicine, summed up five lifestyle components that lead to brain health:

- Physical activity
- Nutrition
- Socialization
- Mental stimulation
- Spirituality

You've read about the first four at length, and you'll find plenty of useful tips at the end of the book on ways to get started in all these areas.

But what does Nussbaum mean by spirituality? He means inner peace—however you can achieve it. Too many people walk around feeling stressed, angry, and frustrated, which has obvious physical effects on cognitive health, as shown in Dr. Bennett's studies on populations of older people.

Inner peace is about becoming just as aware of what's going on inside your body as outside. "We're not so good at that—a heart attack may feel like jaw pain or arm pain," Dr. Nussbaum explains. "We don't have the same sensitivity as we do when we see there's a snake three inches from our leg."

But it is possible to become more in tune with your body's inner signals, once you shut off the faucet of stress. "Whether it's deep prayer or deep meditation ... that seems to bring the brain into an electrical state of stabilization," he says. "It's about how do we think about getting the brain to reduce its stress so that it functions in an efficient way. You'll never maximize mental stimulation, or physical activity, or nutrition unless the brain is in a state where it can do what it does best."

Part 5

Stress, Sleep, and Sex

Stressed Out, Stressed Within

Stress is like a member of my household. Both Jim and I have always had a lot of stress from our jobs, and when you add three kids to the mix, it can get pretty intense.

Running a busy law practice may look like a glamorous occupation on TV, but the fact is, Jim has to be prepared for a huge number of important court dates and trials, manage hundreds of filing deadlines and requirements, be responsive to every client need or problem, and be sensitive to every employee's personal and professional triumph or tribulation. He also has to be sure the practice is strong, no matter what the economy or his personal life might throw at him. Don't get me wrong, he loves the professional accomplishments and client interactions, but it can be grueling—and definitely stressful.

That I've spent years as a reporter chasing stories and deadlines before coming home and chasing kids and bedtimes hasn't exactly lessened the load of stress we bring home to our 112-year-old house with toys on the floor and laundry to be done. But life is also fun and exciting. The challenges and achievements keep us going.

But I have learned that different people deal with stress differently. For example, I sometimes wake up at 4 in the morning and can't go back to sleep. If Jim wakes up at 4 in the morning, he's back in dreamland 5 minutes later, which makes me hate him (at least at 4 in the morning). He has learned how to push aside the stress when he needs to.

Stress made sense as an evolutionary adaptation tens of thousands of years ago when early humans needed to be able to quickly summon tremendous energy and effort to escape life-threatening situations. But today, those same physical reactions are often set in motion by much smaller triggers such as being late for a doctor's appointment or losing your keys. Stress has become a constant companion in modern-day life. It's the way you feel when you have more to do than you think you can get done, which is how many people feel much of the time.

Having a little stress is not a bad thing; it tends to help in difficult situations. The hormones released when you're anxious can quickly mobilize energy stores and make your thoughts highly focused. Performers and athletes find a little nervousness before a show or race can actually improve their performance.

But stress has become the new normal. We're spending more time at work, using electronics, and sitting in traffic, and the result is we feel like we have less time to relax, take care of ourselves, pursue new interests, or just be alone and *think*. Americans today often say they're "too busy" to do many of the activities that could help mitigate their stress, such as exercising, sleeping, reading, socializing, spending time in nature, volunteering, and so on.

Clearly, stress is something you want less of, but it often feels like something you can't change. Maybe it comes from an immutable source, such as caring for an elderly parent, or from a traumatic experience that can't be undone. Or maybe the stress from everyday life has begun to feel sourceless—unrelated to anything but affecting everything, until it feels like it's always there, no matter what you do. When stress gets to that point, it accelerates the aging process.

Instinctively, of course, we know stress isn't good for us, because it just feels bad. But scientists are only just now pinpointing the link

> "Scientists are only just now pinpointing the link between stress and aging and the harm stress poses over the long term."

between stress and aging and the harm stress poses over the long term.

Studies have linked stress to a variety of health problems, including the following:

- A weakened immune system
- Cardiovascular disease
- Stroke
- Inflammation
- Premature cell aging
- Cancer
- Dementia

But stress is something you *can* change, even if the trigger of your stress cannot be removed or identified. Just as scientists are beginning to understand the complex ways stress makes us sick, they're also finding that age-old techniques of stress reduction, which you can learn with just a little guidance, actually have the power to slow down aging.

Physical Feelings

It may not always seem like it, but stress starts out as a psychological phenomenon—a feeling, thought, or emotion. Maybe you're distressed about something you've seen, worried about not getting everything done, or afraid that something bad will happen in the future. When such thoughts come into your head, your body's stress-response system releases various hormones and chemicals in your brain that *convert* those emotions into physical reactions—all designed to protect you in the event of physical harm.

When you experience stress, your body sets in motion a flurry of activities:

- Your breathing and heartbeat rates become rapid, increasing oxygen to your lungs and blood flow to your muscles, giving you the energy boost needed to make a quick getaway.

- Blood flows away from your skin, making you cold and clammy, which will make you bleed less if you're wounded.

- Your digestive system shuts down, suppressing your appetite, because it's not necessary when you're in survival mode.

- Chemicals in your brain suppress activity in areas used for short-term memory, rational thought, inhibition, and concentration.

These are just some of the reactions that can affect you physically during times of stress. When the feeling of fear or worry passes, your physical state returns to normal. Many people cycle in and out of these symptoms regularly, perhaps even unaware of the negative or fearful thought that precipitated the reaction. When it happens all the time, it begins to seem normal.

But it's not. The effect of these stress-related hormones on your cells builds up over time and ages you. In a 2011 interview on radio's *The Dr. Molly Barrow Show,* cell-aging expert Dr. Elissa Epel, psychologist with the University of California, San Francisco, explained the connection with utter clarity: "In a sense, our cells are listening to our thoughts and feelings." When your thoughts and feelings aren't healthy, neither are your cells.

> "When your thoughts and feelings aren't healthy, neither are your cells."

Here are some of the effects stress has on your body in ways you *don't* see or feel:

Decreased immunity: There's a long-standing body of research linking chronic and acute stress with decreased immune system function. Stressed people get more colds and flu and even more cancer. Why this happens isn't well understood, but it is believed that stress hormones interfere with genes and signals that regulate the immune system. Stress has also been found to promote cancerous tumor growth by inhibiting the body's natural antitumor immune response.

Atherosclerosis: The hormone imbalance caused by high levels of circulating stress hormones interferes with the proper function of endothelial cells that line all your veins and arteries. This can lead to hardening of the arteries, or atherosclerosis, a major risk factor for heart disease.

Shorter telomeres: Groundbreaking work in Dr. Epel's lab at the University of California, San Francisco, has linked stress to shorter telomeres, the protective caps at the ends of the chromosomes that protect the genetic code and allow for normal cell division. Shorter telomeres have been found to be a clear marker of cell aging. When telomeres get too short, cells stop dividing, and a buildup of these senescent cells eventually causes tissue malfunction and symptoms associated with aging. Shorter telomeres could also explain the effect of stress on immunity, because immune cells need to multiply quickly to fight infection and invaders. If telomeres are compromised, immune cells may not be able to multiply enough to mount an effective defense.

Hormone imbalance: The many hormones and neurotransmitters released as a result of stress—and there are many—can impact other hormones in the body. These interactions are so complex that they're still not well understood. One example is the effect of cortisol, one of the main stress hormones produced by the adrenal gland, on another adrenal hormone called dehydroepiandrosterone (DHEA). Higher levels of DHEA have been linked to better feelings of well-being, while lower levels have been linked to an increase in frailty in the elderly. If chronic stress is pushing your cortisol levels abnormally high, there's evidence it could suppress DHEA levels, which could have negative health consequences.

Inflammation: Various labs have been trying to explain the link between stress and systemic inflammation, a condition that seems to encourage or worsen a variety of age-related diseases such as heart disease. In trying to establish that individuals under high stress have higher levels of inflammation, Carnegie Mellon University social psychologist Dr. Sheldon Cohen, who studies the impact of stress on health, used the cold virus to detect existing inflammation in stressed individuals. He chose this approach because the symptoms of a cold do not come from the virus itself, but from the inflammation caused by the body's immune response to the virus.

In Dr. Cohen's study, published in 2012 in the *Proceedings of the National Academy of Sciences,* Cohen exposed 276 healthy adults to a cold virus and then monitored them in quarantine for 5 days. The subjects who developed the most severe cold symptoms were those who had previously experienced a prolonged stressful event. Because their inflammatory systems were already heightened from stress, Cohen concluded, they were more likely to develop severe cold symptoms from the additional immune-related inflammation.

Brain size: Increased levels of stress, post-traumatic stress disorder, and high levels of cortisol in the blood have all been linked to a smaller hippocampus, a critical region of the brain that is responsible for encoding much of what we experience. This is the first region of the brain to lose functionality in Alzheimer's disease. It's still unclear if someone with a smaller hippocampus is more susceptible to stress, or if stress leads to shrinkage of the hippocampus. But a recent 32-year population study of women who developed brain atrophy later in life found a direct correlation between atrophy and increased frequency of severe psychological distress.

It Happens in the Hippocampus

For such a tiny structure, the hippocampus is incredibly powerful. It records what we experience in our lives and lays it down as short- and long-term memories—or discards what we don't need to remember. It's also responsible for spatial navigation. The hippocampus is usually the first area of the brain to show damage from dementia, which shows up as memory problems and disorientation. That could be because the hippocampus is uniquely responsive to the life you lead: it has high levels of receptors for stress hormones, such as cortisol, making it especially vulnerable to long-term stress. But it's also one of the few areas of the brain that's been proven to be capable of neurogenesis, or growing of new neurons, in response to such beneficial behaviors as learning new things and exercise.

If you weren't already convinced, you should be now: stress is bad for you. It feels bad, it's exhausting, and it ages you all the way down to your cells.

The Future Factor

It is possible to limit the physical effects of stress without resorting to medication, but doing so requires a little bit of rethinking—literally.

The only way to stop the cascade of harmful hormones that flow through your body as a result of stress is to stop them before they start. And the only way to do that is to control the thoughts that trigger the stress response. This is what Jim does so successfully at 4 in the morning if he happens to wake up.

But it wasn't always like that. We used to both toss and turn if we happened to wake up at the same time, but at some point, it changed—for him. When I asked Jim how he managed to go back to sleep, he said, "I just decided that whatever it is I'm worried about I can't fix at 4 in the morning anyway, so I started forcing myself to think about something else. Then I just fall asleep."

> "When I asked Jim how he managed to go back to sleep, he said, 'I just decided that whatever it is I'm worried about I can't fix at 4 in the morning anyway.'"

I tried that, and it rarely worked for me, maybe because I didn't get enough practice because it only happens once or twice a week. But I think the problem is that I wasn't trying hard enough. Several studies on meditation and deep breathing convinced me to try harder—and to reject my inner doubt it could possibly work for me. It took a couple weeks of concentrated effort (at 4 in the morning!) to force myself to think about just one thing rather than everything else my mind wanted to think about. It's now been 3 months since I've woken up in the night and not been able to go back to sleep—even on nights when I felt overwhelmed by impending book deadlines, camp inquiries I hadn't made, airplane reservations I hadn't had time to book, laundry I hadn't done, and so on.

Dr. Aiofe O'Donovan, PhD, psychologist and stress researcher in Elissa Epel's lab at the University of California, San Francisco, calls this kind of diversion tactic "attentional control" and considers it an "incredible skill." When we're stuck in a cycle of stress, it's easy to get mired in negative, disastrous thoughts. For me, that cycle has always been a familiar one: *Uh-oh, I'm awake at 4 in the morning. If I don't go back to sleep I'm going to feel lousy today. If I feel terrible today, I won't be able to get everything done I need to get done.* Which, of course, only means I feel more anxious and become even less likely to go back to sleep.

Dr. O'Donovan's latest studies suggest that people who have the ability to make themselves stop worrying, or decide to worry at a later time, actually have longer telomeres. Unfortunately, the opposite is also true. In a recent study, O'Donovan gave two stress-provoking tasks to a group of about 50 women, half of whom were chronically stressed from caring for a relative with dementia. The women were given a public speaking assignment and asked to perform complex math calculations (successively subtracting 17 from a large number) in front of others, without a calculator. The women were told ahead of time what they would have to do and asked how they felt about it.

O'Donovan says the women who were chronically stressed caregivers generally felt more "threatened" (a term used in the study to measure more substantive feelings than everyday anxiety) by the upcoming event than the women who were not caregivers. And the caregivers who felt the *most* threatened by the upcoming performance turned out to have the shortest telomeres, meaning their cells showed the signs of accelerated aging.

"This told us that it's this long-term anticipation of stress that could be having the biggest effect," Dr. O'Donovan explains. "One of the major things about being human is we can imagine the future and we can predict the future. It allows us to control our environment and plan and make choices based on our future ideal. But it also allows us to activate our stress response far in advance of a real stressor. When we activate that response weeks or months in advance, we put our bodies through excess preparation and we activate these responses to the point that they become harmful."

Once again, here's a human behavior that was useful through our evolution because it made us better able to predict danger and, therefore, avoid it, but that is now out of place in today's relatively safe and stable world.

Another adaptation that can be harmful is that stress tends to build on itself, O'Donovan says, so if you're stressed, you become more sensitive to new stress. This also made sense from an evolutionary perspective because if an ancient human was threatened by a fierce animal, he would have a greater chance of surviving if he stayed on alert for new threats from that predator or others that might be nearby.

Today, that adaptation means that if you're already feeling stressed about a deadline at work and then misplace your keys, you'll have a much stronger negative response than you would have if you had been in a calm state of mind when you realized your keys were missing. "The small stressful things that happen to us in life become more threatening against a backdrop of chronic stress," says O'Donovan.

Psychologists who study aging suggest several ways to reduce the impact of stress on your physical health, including exercise, controlling your thoughts, and sleep. I explain the overwhelming importance of sleep and how much it affects the way you age at length in the next chapter, but let's look at how some other widely studied approaches to alleviating stress appear to work.

> "'The small stressful things that happen to us in life become more threatening against a backdrop of chronic stress.'"

Cognitive Therapy

This well-established discipline is aimed at noticing and stopping dysfunctional, negative thoughts and changing them to something more rational or positive. If you can adjust your thinking, you can dampen the trigger of your stress response and lessen your physical reaction to it. An example might be catching yourself feeling extremely stressed because you're running late to an appointment. Here's what cognitive therapy would have you do:

1. Identify what it is that's making you feel stressed.

2. Make a list—in your head or on paper—of the reasons that being late is upsetting you, such as:

    I might miss my appointment if the doctor can't squeeze me in.

    I will be late for my next appointment.

    It will make the doctor angry.

    I will inconvenience other patients.

3. Challenge each item on your list with a more rational thought. In this case, you might think:

    Doctors always try to squeeze in patients.

    I can let them know I have somewhere else to be, and I can call my other appointment to let them know I'll be late.

    Doctors know some patients will be late, so they aren't likely to get angry when it happens.

    Doctors build time into their schedules for things to get backed up, so it's not likely to hurt anyone else, or at least not much.

This ritual seems almost too simple to work, but it's remarkably effective because the thoughts that send us into a stressed state are *automatic thoughts* that are *not rational*. These thoughts are generated not by your conscious brain, with all its experience and wisdom, but by the prehistoric emotional center of your brain that still reacts to anxiety as though you are in mortal danger. But by suppressing your automatic thoughts with more rational ones based on real-life experience, you can control your emotional response.

This is a fundamental life skill, according to Dr. Daniel Amen, well-known psychiatrist and prolific author of numerous books on brain health. The principles of cognitive therapy, he says, are life-changing, even in children. Yet most of us grow up unable to challenge—much less dismiss—our own thoughts. We don't even know it's possible. "Nowhere in school does our system teach kids not to believe every stupid thought they have," Amen says. "You have to get sick and go to the psychologist before someone teaches you cognitive therapy. They should be teaching cognitive therapy to kindergarteners."

Although this technique is often used to treat depression and panic disorder, you can try it yourself to help minimize the effects of stress, chronic or acute. It feels a little awkward at first, but eventually you'll learn to instantly challenge your automatic thoughts so your stress levels go down. If you can reduce the flow of stress hormones into your body, you'll not only feel better, you'll be healthier in the long run.

Exercise

In case you haven't seen enough evidence yet that exercise can help you age less, here's another reason to get up and move: exercise reduces the effects of stress.

Many studies have demonstrated this relationship in both humans and animals, although exactly how exercise has these stress-busting effects is less clear. One possibility is that exercise stimulates the release of various chemicals that make you feel good and block the effects of stress hormones. Neurotransmitters called endorphins that are released during exercise, for example, block pain receptors in the brain and promote feelings of well-being—and not just because you're proud of yourself for exercising!

Other scientists have suggested that the physical demands of exercise force the body's energy, cardiovascular system, and endocrine (hormone) system to coordinate precisely and, as a result, become more finely tuned, leading to fewer out-of-whack signals and responses.

Physical activity helps counteract the telomere-shortening effects of stress. People who exercise have been found to have longer telomeres.

Many Americans exercise to lose weight and look better in a bathing suit. But exercise has so many more benefits that are easier to achieve. When you exercise, you feel happier, stress less, sleep better, minimize free radical damage, have better immune function, and have longer telomeres. It doesn't take as much exercise to reap those rewards as it would to reshape your body, so even if you can't keep up with the amount of exercise you need to make a difference in the way you look, don't let that keep you from exercising. Instead, keep at it for all the reasons you *can't* see: not so much as a way to *look* good, but as a way to *feel* good and age less.

> "Even if you can't keep up with the amount of exercise you need to make a difference in the way you look, don't let that keep you from exercising. Instead, keep at it for all the reasons you *can't* see."

Meditation, Mindfulness, and Relaxation

These practices are somewhat related to cognitive therapy, in that they involve altering your patterns of thought, but they operate, and are beneficial, in a different way. All three have been shown to have clear psychological benefits and even cause beneficial structural changes in the brain. Talk about a mind-body connection!

Mindfulness: This is often referred to as "living in the moment." Being more mindful means making an effort to be aware of everything you do at the moment you're doing it and noticing how your actions and motivations work together.

On a daily basis, being more mindful means devoting all your attention to what you're doing at that time, so you're *not* texting while you're at the dinner table, and you're *not* looking around the room while you're talking to someone. It is, truly, the opposite of multitasking.

The benefit of mindfulness is that negative, stress-causing emotions usually don't come from what's happening at that moment but from thoughts related to the past or the future. By focusing only on what's going on immediately around you at any given point in time, your mind will get a break from the thoughts that lead to stress, giving your cells a chance to rest and recover from the damage stress brings.

But mindfulness has a broader usefulness, too. It gives you a better understanding of what's happening, why, and how you're a part of it. So if it's your goal to eat more fruits and vegetables, for example, try to be more mindful about noticing opportunities when you could add a fruit snack or eat another vegetable with dinner. Especially when we're stressed, we tend to miss out on opportunities to make easy changes that could help ease our stress.

To really practice the art of mindfulness and achieve greater control of your emotions and actions, aim for these tactics:

- Remind yourself what really matters to you: is a decision you've made going to help you reach that goal?
- Be aware of what you're doing: are you mindlessly surfing the internet rather than getting that project done?
- Notice when you're making decisions: are your decisions making a problem worse or preventing you from feeling better?
- Pay attention to what's happening when things go wrong: look for patterns in your decisions, such as noticing if you tend to make bad decisions when you're tired or stressed.

Mindfulness is not always easy, especially in the beginning. But you can start small. Try it anytime, anywhere. To get started, try this:

- Fully listen to someone, without thinking about anything else while you do so.
- Watch your kids play without picking up your phone.
- Talk to your spouse when you're not doing something else at the same time, such as watching TV or making dinner.

- Listen with all your focus in a meeting, or watch TV without checking your email.
- Watch the sun set, and think only about the sunset. Don't let your mind wander!

Mindful Eating

The next time you eat, pay attention to the way food feels, tastes, and sounds as you chew it. When you learn to really appreciate your food, it will help control your cravings and better regulate your hunger. You can also pay attention not just to the food, but to the experiences you create with food, noticing the choices you make and tying those decisions to your motivations. Are you eating for energy? For taste? Are you serving food to entertain friends? Establish a goal for what and how you eat, and make choices consistent with that goal. It may take time to approach food this way, but with time, it will get easier!

Mindfulness does more than just shut off stressful thoughts for a moment; it can become second nature. It's a skill like anything else, and as you get better at it, you get better at controlling your stress. You may not believe it, but it really works.

In a recent study conducted by researchers at the University of Kentucky and published in the *Journal of Clinical Psychology*, 87 adults with high levels of chronic stress went through an 8-week program of mindfulness training. The participants assessed their own mindfulness skills and their level of perceived stress each week. After 2 weeks, subjects showed significant increases in mindfulness. And after 4 weeks, they showed "significant improvements" in perceived stress, the researchers reported.

Meditation: Meditation has many different forms, but mindfulness is a key component of most of them. Unlike everyday mindfulness, meditation usually involves focusing on something in particular, such as your breathing, and training your mind not to wander as you focus on that one thing. During meditation, for example, you might focus only on the feeling of your breath going into your body, how it feels passing through your nostrils and expanding your diaphragm. This is the "attentional control" skill O'Donovan mentions as so valuable, and it's what Jim does at 4 in the morning, even if he doesn't meditate the rest of the day.

As a novice meditator, it's hard at first to keep your thoughts from migrating away to other sounds, feelings, or memories, which is why it takes a while for meditation to begin working on stress. But over time, like a muscle that gets trained, the brain actually becomes better able to screen out distractions and focus on what you want to focus on. It gets so much better, it can be seen on an MRI.

Attentional control is regulated by specific regions of the brain that, when observed on an MRI, light up during meditation exercises. Over time, that kind of focused activity actually builds brain tissue in those areas, which gives you greater ability to perform that kind of task. You get better at meditating the more you do it because you're growing new brain cells just for that purpose.

> "Over time, like a muscle that gets trained, the brain actually becomes better able to screen out distractions and focus on what you want to focus on. It gets so much better, it can be seen on an MRI."

A study conducted by researchers at Massachusetts General Hospital, and published in 2011 in the journal *Psychiatry Research: Neuroimaging,* studied the brain structure of 16 participants by MRI both before and after doing an 8-week mindfulness-meditation training program. The MRI studies at the end of the program found that the brain structures that control self-awareness, compassion, introspection, learning, and memory had all increased in size. At the same time, though, the density of gray matter decreased in the areas of the brain associated with stress and anxiety. These two opposing changes correlated with reductions in stress reported by the participants.

Members of the control group in this study, who did not participate in the meditation training, showed no such structural changes in their brains and no change in their stress levels.

Clock-Cheater Tip

Meditation is worth a try, whether you take a class or try it at home. Expect a training period of about 4 weeks, during which you take just a few minutes each day, or as often as you can, to meditate. Try 5 minutes before bed or when you first wake up. Turn off all distractions, and try to empty your mind. Notice when stray thoughts pop into your head, and push them away. It can be helpful to visualize something or repeat a phrase. It will be frustrating at first, but it will get easier! You'll eventually build new neurons in your brain that have one special skill: keeping you calm and managing your stress.

It's a powerful thing to be able to rewire your brain. Indeed, some studies have even shown greater reductions in self-reported stress from meditation work than from either aerobic physical activity or cognitive therapy.

Relaxation: Sometimes all it takes to stop stress-inducing thoughts is to use a few quick relaxation techniques, such as simple deep breathing, using slow, deep, purposeful breaths. Even if you're feeling stressed, deep breathing helps your brain shut down your anxious, threatened feelings and responses.

"Deep breathing is very, very powerful," explains Dr. Paul Nussbaum, neuropsychologist and adjunct professor at the University of Pittsburgh School of Medicine. "It shuts down the sympathetic nervous system and sets off the parasympathetic nervous system."

The sympathetic and parasympathetic nervous systems are both part of the autonomic nervous system, which unconsciously regulates all your internal organs and systems. The sympathetic nervous system is responsible for stimulation associated with the fight-or-flight response. The parasympathetic nervous system, meanwhile, controls rest-and-digest activities. Deep breathing activates a more restful and calming cascade of signals from the brain.

Visualizing something beautiful and peaceful has a similar effect. It works especially well if you can incorporate as many of your senses as possible. For example, if you visualize yourself in a forest, try to smell the moss, hear the birds, and feel the crunching leaves underfoot.

Other well-known ways to relax have been shown to help stress levels, including massage, yoga, or even just sitting in a warm bath. It's not self-indulgent; it's self-preservation.

The goal of all these approaches is to take your mind away from the thoughts and emotions that lead to stress. These techniques are all drug-free tools you can use to turn your thoughts away from the fearful, anxious feelings that, over time, accelerate aging. You may not be able to get rid of the original cause of your stress, but that's all the more reason to learn better techniques for managing it, so your stress level is less toxic to your cells. As Dr. O'Donovan's studies have shown, it's not the stress-inducing event, person, or problem that harms your health long term; it's how you handle it.

The Significance of Sleep

You already know my husband, Jim, has a remarkable ability to make himself go back to sleep in the middle of the night rather than lie there worrying about things. Clearly he possesses powerful thought-diverting skills, but he also has an innate appreciation of sleep that many people don't—or that they ignore, as I often do. It's not that I'm a night owl; it's that I get backed up during the day and then at 11 P.M. I make a conscious decision to stay up longer to get a few things done that I had wanted to accomplish earlier in the day, such as emails, or looking over a school project, or just some more writing.

And when I do that, Jim invariably walks by me and says something like, "You'll get more done if you go to bed and do it in the morning."

Jim tries very hard to get at least 7 hours of sleep a night. It's not always possible, of course. Sometimes just getting to bed by 11:30 seems like a Herculean effort, given the lingering demands of work, taking care of the house, three kids, and the school projects they seem to "remember" the night before they're due. Yet the 6 A.M. alarm clock, and the school bell, are immutable. (All of which leads me to suggest that kids are a risk factor for aging, but at least they'll be there to take care of you when they've made you old. Or at least they better!)

Unlike many people, Jim actually thinks about the effect of sleep on his performance. He's in tune with the way he feels, and he recognizes that when he doesn't get enough sleep, he simply can't function at the level he needs to in order to get his work done effectively and still be helpful at night. "Everything's better when you get a good night's sleep," he says (and says, and says). So if he has gone 2 or 3 days getting only 6 or 6¹/₂ hours of shut-eye, stay out of his way at 10:30 because come hell or high water, he will be asleep at 11 P.M. Could this be another discipline that's helping him age so well? Considering the science, the answer is most likely "yes."

> "He recognizes that when he doesn't get enough sleep, he simply can't function at the level he needs to in order to get his work done effectively."

We spend a third of our lives sleeping, and scientists and researchers have been studying sleep for decades, if not hundreds of years, yet we still don't really know why or even how we do it. But they are beginning to understand the long-term health consequences of not getting enough sleep.

Sleep and aging are closely connected. Older people don't sleep as well as younger people, and scientists are beginning to find evidence of a vicious cycle: not sleeping well leads to aging, and aging leads to not sleeping well.

People with chronic sleep problems are at much higher risk of a host of diseases and conditions usually considered age-related, including diabetes, dementia, and hypertension. They gain weight more easily and are more susceptible to general illness, less responsive to vaccines, more vulnerable to stress and depression, and tend to have higher blood pressure. Now, perhaps not surprisingly, researchers have linked markers of accelerated cellular aging to poor sleep. Your cells, once again, are listening.

Yet getting too little sleep has become a major problem in this country. About 10 percent of the population suffer from true insomnia, and a quarter reports occasional sleep problems, according to the Centers for Disease Control. Some people suffering from true medical or hormonal conditions that interfere with sleep may find varying degrees of help from behavioral and medical interventions, such as meditation (again) or sleeping pills.

But the real problem seems to be, increasingly, that we just don't seem to value sleep enough. We power through until late at night, ignoring our body's sleep signals as we hammer on the computer or otherwise work (or play) until the wee hours. If we sleep a little less, so what? We're getting it done and getting ahead! Sleep data suggests this is the trend. Thirty years ago, time-use studies conducted by the government showed that the typical American got just over 8 hours of sleep. In 2007, the same study showed Americans get just over 7 hours of sleep a night.

You may see that and think, *One hour less sleep. What's the big deal?* But 1 hour is a big deal when you start to get below 7 hours of sleep. And if the average American gets 7 hours, a whole lot of people are getting a lot less than that average.

Immunity Mutiny and More

Although sleep deficits appear to influence and speed up the aging process over time, the impact of sleeping just a little bit less can be immediate.

Remember Carnegie Mellon researcher Sheldon Cohen, who tested for inflammation in stressed individuals by exposing them to the cold virus? Well, he seems to make a habit of exposing subjects to cold viruses: in another study, he used the rhinovirus to see if people who sleep less are more vulnerable to the common cold.

His team tracked the sleep habits of 153 healthy adults age 21 to 55 for 2 weeks and then exposed each of them to the common cold by putting droplets of the virus in their nostrils and quarantined them in a hotel for 5 days. Nearly 90 percent of the subjects became infected with the virus—that is, it started replicating inside their bodies. But only 54 individuals developed actual cold symptoms. And who were those people? The ones who slept the least.

Once all the data were tallied, the study showed that people who slept less than 7 hours a night were three times more likely to develop cold symptoms than people who averaged 8 or more hours of sleep a night. And subjects whose sleep was disturbed or broken up fared even worse: subjects who reported spending more than 8 percent of their time in bed tossing and turning had a nearly six-fold greater risk of developing a cold (called sleep efficiency). The study, which was reported in the *Archives of Internal Medicine* in 2012, is thought to be the first to show that such a small sleep deficit can compromise the immune system.

> "People who slept less than 7 hours a night were three times more likely to develop cold symptoms."

And if you regularly forgo some sleep because you feel okay even without a full 8 hours, consider this: Cohen found that "feeling rested" was not protective. The only measures that mattered in preventing infection were getting more than 7 hours and sleeping efficiently.

Dr. Cohen's study is a wake-up call about the impact sleep has on our day-to-day health. But the bigger problem with lack of sleep is looming years down the road, thanks to all the ways sleep deficits build up in your body and slowly erode your health and vitality. At some point, you just may wonder if all those late nights with Jay Leno and Facebook were really worth it.

Another study looking at the difference in getting just an hour or two less sleep found that people who slept the least had the greatest buildup of calcium in their arteries—a known precursor to heart disease—5 years later. Nearly 500 people age 35 to 47 participated in the study, conducted at the University of Chicago Medical Center. They wore wristbands to measure sleep and had CT scans before and after the study to measure calcium buildup in their arteries.

Over the 5 years, artery calcification was detected in 27 percent of the subjects who slept 5 hours a night, but in only 6 percent of those who slept 7 hours a night. The study authors believe the results may stem from the fact that blood pressure falls when sleeping, so more sleep means more time in each 24-hour period with low blood pressure.

Maybe the chance of developing heart disease years from now won't get you to shut off the tube or computer and get some shut-eye tonight. But how about getting fat? Would that do it? Numerous studies have found that people who don't get enough sleep tend to be heavier. You might have noticed this yourself. When you don't sleep well, you're often hungrier the next day; crave sugary, fatty foods; and don't get the feeling of being satisfied.

If so, you're not alone. A study published in *The American Journal of Clinical Nutrition* in 2011 observed that sleep-deprived subjects consumed, on average, 300 more calories a day. A study conducted at the Mayo Clinic found that being restricted to two thirds of their usual sleep time made people eat an average of 549 extra calories a day! Still another study done at Brigham and Women's Hospital and published in 2012 found that subjects whose sleep patterns were not only shortened but also moved around in a 24-hour period, to mimic jet lag or variable work shifts, showed decline in metabolic rate big enough to cause a 10- to 12-pound weight gain in a year.

"Artery calcification was detected in 27 percent of the subjects who slept 5 hours a night, but in only 6 percent of those who slept 7 hours a night."

If scientists don't know why we sleep, or how we sleep, do they at least know why *not* sleeping makes us eat more? The mechanism underpinning this unfortunate relationship appears to be hormonal.

Several studies have shown that lack of sleep raises the production of ghrelin, a hormone produced in the digestive tract that's responsible for making you feel hungry. At the same time, poor sleep lowers levels of leptin, a hormone made by fat cells that tells you when you're full and gives you a feeling of satisfaction with what you've eaten. These are complicated signals to figure out, and the research is far from clear. But whatever the underlying reason, the science is abundantly clear that if you don't sleep enough, you're likely to eat more, eat worse foods, and gain weight.

It should come as no surprise, then, that the University of California, San Francisco, teams who have done so much work measuring telomeres have also found that women with poor sleep habits have—you guessed it—shorter telomeres. What was interesting about this study was that it found the biggest difference in telomere length was related not to the duration of sleep, but to a woman's perception of how well she slept, according to the study's lead author, Dr. Aric Prather. The study adjusted the data to remove the effect of stress, which is known to shorten telomeres, and found poor sleep quality still had an impact on telomere length.

> "The science is abundantly clear that if you don't sleep enough, you're likely to eat more, eat worse foods, and gain weight."

Of course, this study provides doubly bad news for people with chronic stress, because they are exactly the population who tends to have trouble sleeping, Dr. Prather says.

Problem Sleep: Cause and Cure

There are only theories about why and how we sleep. Scientists know that getting stretches of uninterrupted sleep is critical for solidifying memories, for example. Mice woken up repeatedly can't remember the toys they played with the day before. But obviously, there's something more crucial going on. Sleep is so essential that a rare genetic disorder, appropriately called fatal familial insomnia, eventually robs people of the ability to sleep and results in certain death, usually within a year. Lab animals, too, when deprived of sleep, quickly succumb to one disease or another.

As to what makes us fall asleep, the answers are no clearer. Lemont Kier, professor of medicinal chemistry at Virginia Commonwealth University, has theorized that a buildup of nitrogen in our brains each day from breathing the air around us—which is 78 percent nitrogen—gradually anesthetizes the brain and puts us to sleep. Only after a period of slow, shallow breathing during sleep does the nitrogen dissipate.

With so few concrete answers to fundamental questions about sleep and lots of novel theories, scientists worry that people don't take sleep as seriously as they should. Scientists don't know, for example, why one person needs less sleep than another, but some do. There are even so-called *elite sleepers* who can get by with just 2 or 3 hours of sleep a night and experience no sense of sleep deprivation and no ill health effects. Those people tend to know who they are, but doctors and scientists have no way to test for it. And most people who say they don't "need" 8 hours of sleep probably do; they just power through the feelings of sleepiness, extra hunger, and lack of focus, perhaps assuming that's what "normal" feels like.

But even if we can't figure out what makes us sleep, can we at least figure out what makes us sleep badly? There are some clues, but like the process of aging, it seems to be a complex symphony of factors. For example, scientists have identified a few variants of genes that are associated with poor sleep ability, but that doesn't necessarily mean if you have those genes you won't be able to sleep well. Brain structure also seems to play a role. And other researchers have identified a greater need for sleep when the brain has been exercised through learning new things and having new experiences, which could explain why the elderly often sleep poorly.

And then there are more provocative studies that seem to get at the very nature of being human. As social creatures through the millennia, loneliness appears to be particularly damaging to human health: lack of social connectivity leads to dementia, heart disease, even slow wound healing. Scientists have connected these outcomes to lack of sleep.

A 2011 study published in the journal *Sleep* compared feelings of loneliness to a person's sleep quality in two distinctly different groups: undergraduate college students and members of a South Dakota religious community called the Hutterites. The Hutterites live in close-knit groups of extended families who share every aspect of their lives with one another, from work to meals to religious observance.

Despite that social closeness, though, some Hutterites still express feelings of loneliness. So do some college students, obviously. There simply are some people who have difficulty feeling satisfied with their social connections, no matter what their level of social interaction. The significant finding in the study was that for both the Hutterites and the college students, despite living in vastly different lifestyles, those who felt the loneliest were the people who experienced the most fragmented sleep.

The authors of the study suggest that this fragmented sleep, known to cause major health problems, could be the mechanism that makes loneliness or depression affect someone's health. In other words, maybe it's not the loneliness itself that leads to poor health outcomes, but the poor sleep quality common among those who suffer from such psychological distress.

> "Maybe it's not the loneliness itself that leads to poor health outcomes, but the poor sleep quality common among those who suffer from such psychological distress."

The science that seems to hold the most promise for the sleepless is the study of sleep solutions. People simply need more sleep. Forget about *why* they do, and figure out how they can *get* it.

Sleep disturbances come in many forms: insomnia; sleep apnea (constant waking due to interrupted breathing and low oxygen levels); interrupted sleep from frequent or prolonged awakenings; perceived poor sleep quality, or not feeling "rested" after sleep; daytime sleepiness; and more.

There is no one answer for all these ills, but a few things come close, such as exercise and limiting activities such as working, emailing, eating or drinking, and exercising before bed. Stress-reduction exercises, such as cognitive therapy, meditation, and relaxation techniques, have also been shown in studies to help even chronically bad sleepers get more sleep.

But it can become a vicious cycle: when you don't sleep well, you don't have the willpower or motivation to exercise or take care of yourself, so you sleep less and then get further entrenched in bad habits. The good news is, according to research psychologist Aric Prather of UCSF, "it's one of the few health behaviors that people want to do more of. You get pleasure from it, so it's a little easier to get someone motivated."

Dr. Prather and other sleep specialists suggest that many normal, healthy people who may think they have a medical sleep problem actually have a more conventional sleep problem, which is that they're stuck in a cycle of too little sleep, low motivation, high stress, poor presleep behaviors, and the possible use of sleep medications that can be addictive.

It may seem insurmountable, but if you haven't been diagnosed with a genuine sleep disorder, such as obstructive sleep apnea, you can start making an effort to break the cycle of viewing sleep as a second-rate activity. Making it a priority should become your priority. If you tend to stay up late to get a little extra work done, remember, scientists have proved that a good night's sleep will make you more focused and productive the next day, and that's the best way to get more work done. With every good night's sleep you're also building your brain's defenses against dementia, regulating your diet, becoming happier, and, most likely, prolonging your life.

Shutting your eyes and shutting down for at least 7 hours a night is not a short-term need to get you through the next day; it's a long-term requirement to get you through the full span of your life.

Energy from Intimacy

While you're spending more time between the sheets, there's something else you can do to help your health and put more time on your clock. Here's a hint: it's aerobic, social, enjoyable (or should be), and good for you.

Scientific studies on sex tend to focus on societal issues, like teen sex or attitudes about sex, or physical problems, such as erectile dysfunction, pain during sex, or sex after menopause. But a few scientists have studied the outright benefits of sex and found that just about every aspect of a vibrant sexual relationship is good for both short- and long-term health. The cuddling, the shared experience, the hormones—all of it can make you happier and less stressed, which are key components to a longer life. It's another reason to go to bed early!

This is true around the world. Although many countries, including the United States, have more people living alone now than ever before, the science suggests that a good sex life, when possible, is good for you, no matter what the culture. University of Chicago sociologist Edward O. Laumann conducted a large international survey on the sex lives of men and women over the age of 40 in 29 countries—an enormous effort. The survey, published in 2006 in *Archives of Sexual Behavior,* looked at sexual well-being, a measurement Dr. Laumann used to tie together four distinct issues the survey tracked:

- How respondents rated their physical satisfaction with their sexual relationships
- Their own emotional satisfaction
- Their satisfaction with their own sexual health
- The level of importance of sex in their lives

In every country, the report says, "all four aspects of sexual well-being were significantly related to overall happiness."

"Put *That* in Your Book"

When your sex life is good, you feel it. But like a lot of couples, my husband and I go through periods of having sex more and less frequently, typically tied to job demands, general busy-ness, and stress. Shortly after having our first child, for example, I began working on an early morning television news show for *The Washington Post* and had to go to work at 3:30 in the morning. I had to go to bed every night at 7:30 (often before Jim got home from work) and then got home from work just as he was leaving for the office. I did that job for 3 years, and it was exciting, challenging, and fun.

But it's also why there's a 4-year age difference between our first and second children: we were almost never awake in bed at the same time. Undoubtedly, the lack of sleep, lack of adult companionship, and having a new baby contributed to it, but this was a stressful period in our lives, and I'm sure having almost no opportunity for intimacy contributed to the overall difficulty.

We made an effort to get back on track, and while we still have three kids, two jobs, and a house to look after, we work hard to set aside "alone" time. It's not always easy, of course, but we're both aware that it's important: when we let sex slip for a while, we don't feel as connected, are less relaxed, and more on edge. One recent Saturday night after a particularly aerobic performance, Jim fell back on the bed and said, "Put *that* in your book."

And he's right. Having regular sex has a number of health benefits, the most obvious being that it reduces stress. You feel that, instinctively, but it's actually measurable, and lasting. Dr. Stuart Brody, professor of psychology at the University of West Scotland (Paisley), tracked the sexual behavior of 24 women and 22 men over 2 weeks and then put them through a stressful laboratory experience—again, public speaking and math tests. It turned out the subjects who had engaged in actual intercourse (but not other kinds of sex) during the 2-week period were less stressed in the lab; their blood pressure rose less and recovered faster than people who had not had intercourse. Brody's results were published in the journal *Biological Psychology* in 2006.

Other studies have suggested that people who have intercourse feel less stressed because of the hormone oxytocin, the principal hormone released during sex. Oxytocin—which is also activated by a loving social bond between two partners, between a parent and child, and even by some food such as chocolate—acts on many centers in the brain to suppress anxiety and produce a more social outlook. Several studies have shown that laboratory animals exposed to oxytocin exhibit more positive social behavior and better stress regulation.

Researchers at the Harvard School of Public Health recently tested oxytocin nasal spray on people, and although they found somewhat differing responses between men and women, the subjects who received the oxytocin generally responded better when exposed to a stressful social situation. Results of that study were published in 2012, also in *Biological Psychology*.

Other researchers have looked at the benefits of sex in a variety of ways. Dr. Carl Charnetski, professor of psychology at Wilkes University in Pennsylvania, found that college students who had sex one or two times a week had higher levels of an important antibody, immunoglobulin A, in their saliva.

In addition, two studies analyzed the data gathered from a group of 918 men from Caerphilly, Wales, in the 1980s, including sexual frequency, and followed up to compare with mortality rates. One study found that a man who had sex two or more times a week had a lower risk of a fatal heart attack than men who had sex less than once a month. Another study found that men who had sex two or more times a week had a significant reduction in the risk of death from any cause after 10 years.

And neuropsychologist David Weeks asserted in his 1999 book, *Secrets of the Superyoung*, that having frequent sex can make you look younger. Weeks reported on a study he conducted, showing that men and women who have sex three or four times a week look 10 years younger than people who don't. I don't know about the veracity of his scientific conclusions, but I can tell you, categorically, that this is not a factor in why Jim looks so young.

However, looking younger, having a more active immune system, and feeling less stress could all be related to yet another benefit scientists have linked to a healthy sex life: better sleep. Studies have shown that the feelings of closeness created by oxytocin encourage sleep—and who hasn't pleasantly dozed off after a warm romp with a partner? Researchers believe this may be an evolutionary adaptation from many thousands of years ago, when ancient humans slept huddled together in groups to keep warm and protect themselves from predators. Physical closeness, the release of oxytocin, and sleep became inextricably linked.

> "Weeks reported ... that men and women who have sex three or four times a week look 10 years younger than people who don't."

Emotional Aging

The bonding effect of sex, and sex hormones such as oxytocin and dopamine, is beneficial to your health for the same reason social interaction is. Oxytocin helps people bond and feel safe, and humans thrive when they have a sense of personal connection. Numerous studies have shown that people who don't have it, for whatever reason, are more vulnerable to illness, dementia, and death.

Part of what makes oxytocin so powerful is that it's not released by sex alone, but also by touching and cuddling. It helps mothers and infants bond and reinforces the strong feelings of connection when a couple first falls in love. In the lab, men exposed to oxytocin recall more positive words in relation to the subject of intimate relationships than men who were not exposed to oxytocin, suggesting the hormone plays a role in helping men act loving toward their partners. This also means that relationships with a healthy sexual component, or at least regular physical closeness, will likely be a more loving relationship overall, which is a major benefit for long-term health. This particular study, published in 2008 in *Psychological Science*, was only performed on men, but ask any woman how she feels about cuddling and closeness after sex, and the effect seems pretty obvious!

Understanding the important role that hormones play, not just in sexual attraction but also in general feelings of love and bonding, can make a big difference to a relationship. For example, women often want more hugs and cuddling from a mate before sex: this activity creates a safe, loving, bonded feeling because the physical closeness stimulates the release of oxytocin in her brain. That, in turn, stimulates her desire.

But these feelings of intimacy are also good for your health, because they reduce stress and blood pressure—both of which can help you age better. It can be as simple as holding hands.

In a study done by researchers at the University of North Carolina, two groups of subjects were told they would have to give a public speech. One group sat with their partners holding hands and then embraced for 20 seconds before going on-stage. The other group of couples sat separated from each other. While giving their speeches, the heart rates and blood pressure of subjects in the second group, separated from their partners, rose twice as high as the group who had held hands before performing. If you've ever seen an elderly couple walking down the street holding hands, you know they've got it figured out!

Think about how it feels to fall in love—to be in love. How much better would it be to always feel that way? It would make you feel younger and happier throughout your life. Couples may get used to each other through the years, but making a purposeful effort to do more hand-holding, hugging, and cuddling helps keep hormones flowing so feelings of closeness and warmth keep going strong.

Part 6

Happiness and Well-Being

Happy with Your Hobby

Scientists have found compelling evidence that nurturing your sense of inner peace is a powerful way to reduce stress. People who seem to have that kind of inner balance aren't just born that way, though; they have to work at it. It's a skill to push negative thoughts out of your head and live in the moment. You have to train yourself to appreciate what's good in your life and stop worrying about what's not when you don't have to. But it's a skill anyone can acquire, at any age, using tools readily at your disposal, such as better sleep, meditation, relaxation, friendship, and intimacy.

These peaceful, emotion-centered activities aren't the only way to relieve stress and reduce its age-accelerating effects, however. You can also engage in a compelling diversion or a hobby.

Yes, scientists have found that having a hobby is good for your long-term health—physically and mentally—and can make you age more slowly. Whether it's collecting, gardening, volunteering, cooking, or something else entirely, a hobby diverts your attention away from stressful experiences and thoughts, which reduces the flow of harmful stress hormones to your cells. It gives you a pleasurable reason to interact with people, which increases your social engagement, further reducing your stress, and exercising your brain. And it makes you concentrate, focus, and learn new things, which pushes your brain to make new connections and maintain better cognitive reserve.

It seems so simple that having a hobby can help you age well, but the science is clear: if you find something you enjoy doing and stick with it throughout your life, you are increasing your chances of staying healthy and living longer.

> "If you find something you enjoy doing and stick with it throughout your life, you are increasing your chances of staying healthy and living longer."

A great example of this can be seen in the volunteer program AARP Experience Corps, which started in 1995 as an independent nonprofit with a pilot program in five cities but has since expanded. The goal is to employ retired people age 55 and older to tutor and mentor kids in inner-city schools. Volunteers are asked to contribute at least 15 hours a week, for which they receive a small stipend of about $100 a week.

Initially, the program was aimed at benefitting students and schools, which it does. Students in Experience Corps schools score significantly better on reading tests, the schools report better overall academic achievement, and the school principals deal with fewer discipline problems. But the surprise benefit of the program once it got underway was the enormous health benefits for the volunteers, who have been studied by researchers at Washington University in St. Louis and Johns Hopkins University in Baltimore.

Experience Corps tutors who help kids on a regular basis are less depressed and have greater physical function than retired adults the same age who do not volunteer with the program. But even more striking results came in a study published in 2009 in *The Journal of Gerontology: Medical Sciences*. Dr. Michelle Carson, assistant director of the Center on Aging and Health at Johns Hopkins, used MRI scans and cognitive exams to assess Experience Corps volunteers and found significant changes in their brains as a result of tutoring kids in schools: it actually reversed brain aging in the volunteers.

Of course, this program is aimed at older adults, and not everyone has the time or desire for this kind of commitment. But these studies demonstrate how physically and mentally beneficial a focused, goal-oriented, and social leisure activity can be.

Hobby Healthy

Recently, some of the most interesting research about the benefits of having a hobby has come from scientists in Asia and Europe. For example, researchers in Novi Sad, Serbia, studied the health profile of about 100 female physicians, looking for the variables that were most likely to predict high blood pressure. The study, published in 2010 in the *International Journal of Occupational Environmental Health*, revealed some fairly obvious results, most notably that the biggest factor in making a doctor most susceptible to high blood pressure was exposure to disturbing emotional situations at work, either directly or listening to them.

But what was surprising in the study is that the doctors who were *least* likely to have high blood pressure had three main characteristics: they were the nonsmokers, they had lower body mass indexes, and they had a hobby.

I told a Serbian friend of mine about this study and she laughed. "A hobby?" she asked, incredulous. "That's not the kind of thing you usually hear about Serbia."

It may seem funny at first, the notion of a scrapbooking doctor smiling through the day. But it makes sense. A hobby diverts your mind from work-related stress and connects you with others in a social and nonconfrontational way. That combination lowers your overall stress and blood pressure.

Even more research has been done in Japan, where a trio of studies just in the past couple of years has looked at the beneficial impact of hobbies on long-term health:

Researchers at Ritsumeikan University in Kyoto studied a region in Japan where many of the residents had been recruited to live by the same local employer. The residents of this area have a better

> "A hobby diverts your mind from work-related stress and connects you with others in a social and nonconfrontational way. That combination lowers your overall stress and blood pressure."

health profile than what's seen in Japan generally, so the researchers looked for lifestyle factors that set apart this population. One of the main differences they found is that a high percentage of people in this community participated in organized groups centered on a sport, volunteer activity, or hobby.

A 2012 study out of the University of Tokyo measured the cognitive decline over 5 years in 567 men and women age 70 and older. Above all other variables, including social and physical activity, the results showed that "non-participation in a hobby was significantly and independently associated with cognitive decline."

A study undertaken by the Takamatsu City Public Health Center aimed to describe the health-related quality of life of city residents. This is a measurement used by world health organizations to track factors in life that have a measurable impact on one's physical or mental health. In the Japanese study, researchers looked at the impact of social background, health-related behaviors, and chronic medical conditions in 915 adults. Not surprisingly, they found that the oldest residents, along with those who were stressed, not working, or sick, fared the worst. What made the biggest positive difference? Getting 7 or 8 hours of sleep a night and having a hobby. These two factors, the researchers found, "were significantly associated with increased health-related quality of life."

A Hobby at Home

This research made me look differently at the enormous pleasure my husband gets from photography. It is, undoubtedly, one of the things that sustains Jim through stressful times: put a camera in his hands, and he's off, thinking about something else and brimming with enthusiasm. Getting a single great photograph can take a week's worth of worry off his face.

In fact, photography is the reason we met.

I was working as a hostess in a restaurant during my last year of college, and Jim came in for dinner with a friend, a stylist for a local department store. As she passed by the hostess stand on the way to the ladies room, she stopped me to ask a question. The man she was having dinner with, she explained, was a lawyer who also happened to have an active portrait photography hobby on the side. She was working with him on a photography project for the store, she said. But she also told me this lawyer/photographer had noticed me, and had remarked that he thought I would make a good portrait subject.

The woman had taken it upon herself to ask me if I was interested. "He doesn't know I'm doing this," she said, "but if you'd like to have your portrait taken, I could introduce you on our way out."

So she did, and a couple weeks later, Jim and I met to talk about it. And we just kept talking. In fact, we talked so much, it was months before he took the first picture of me. But even if we had begun to connect on many other levels, I knew right from the start that photography was always going to be part of our relationship, whether I was the subject or not. It was clearly something he was passionate about. Besides me.

Twenty-five years later, we have fabulous and beautiful records of our vacations, our children, our pets, and our house (in every stage of renovation), along with decades of photos that range from photojournalism to fine art. Lately he's been taking pictures of lily pads that don't look like photos at all, but rather paintings.

It is a time-consuming hobby and, especially before digital photography came along, an expensive one. But it's a classic *hobby*, something he does purely for personal pleasure. For a while, he tried taking pictures for hire (like the department store gig), but the responsibility changed the dynamic for him, and it wasn't as much fun. Pursuing photography for himself, however, meant he could enjoy every aspect of it: finding a subject, thinking about it, shooting it, developing it (digitally, now), and, if it turned out to be exceptional, framing it or giving it as a present to a friend or family member. Our house is full of prints, framed and unframed; our shelves stuffed with photography books; our computers packed with digital photo files; our attic overflowing with accessories like studio lamps, background paper, reflectors, tripods, old cameras, and more.

Looking at my husband's face light up (for hours—even days) when he gets a truly fantastic photograph is the only explanation I need to understand these scientific findings. When I was a teenager, I did a lot of knitting, and I remember how I floated around for days when I finished my first sweater made with multiple kinds of stitches and different yarn colors (never mind it turned out to be the *only* sweater of that kind I ever made). That kind of personal satisfaction and sense of accomplishment makes you happy.

And happiness keeps you healthy.

Outlook Matters

Happiness, like good health, is something everyone wants. Because happiness manifests itself both emotionally and physically, it has a huge influence on your life. Happy people don't just feel different from unhappy people; they behave differently and often look better as well.

They even live longer. Researchers at Wayne State University looked at old baseball cards and found that players who were smiling in their photographs had lived longer lives—and the bigger the smile, the longer the life.

The link between happiness and longevity has been shown in many studies, such as an especially compelling one published in the *Archives of Internal Medicine* in 2012, from PhD psychologists Andrew Steptoe and Jane Wardle at University College London. The researchers analyzed data from an aging study on 11,400 men and women in England age 50 and older. They analyzed the subjects' assessed "enjoyment of life," along with various other health and behavior factors, over 7 years. Then they divided the entire study group into four quarters, from the least happy (least life enjoyment) to the most. Then they looked at which of the 1,251 study participants had died during the study period.

Call it the happy effect: subjects with the highest level of life enjoyment had a 57.5 percent reduced risk of death from any cause compared with the lowest enjoyment group.

Of course, someone who has diabetes and a back problem may not enjoy life as much as someone who is perfectly healthy. And that person may die sooner because of that underlying illness. So the researchers had to figure out if unhappiness was contributing to some subjects' death over other factors. To answer that question, they adjusted the data to remove the effects of other conditions potentially related to mortality, including demographics and preexisting health conditions.

Even after making that change, the happy effect persisted and, although lower than the initial measurement, was still striking. When not taking into account illness, low socioeconomic status, and other factors, the people who enjoyed their lives the most still had a 28 percent lower risk of dying compared to those who enjoyed their lives the least.

> "The people who enjoyed their lives the most ... had a 28 percent lower risk of dying compared to those who enjoyed their lives the least."

"These results highlight the importance of positive well-being in older adults and suggest that efforts to improve enjoyment of life ... could have beneficial effects on life expectancy," the authors wrote.

The reason for that effect remains unclear, but scientists are trying to figure it out. Poor sleep is one possible culprit, as suggested by the study on the unhappy Hutterites and the college students. In that study, despite vastly different life experiences, both groups exhibited the same connection between sleep and happiness: those who slept the least well were the most likely to be depressed.

But it could be more complex than that. Aric Prather, the scientist from UCSF who studies sleep and its effect on telomeres, also studies stress and depression. In a study he published in 2012 in the journal *Brain, Behavior, and Immunity,* Dr. Prather found that women who reacted badly to psychological stress in a laboratory experiment also experienced an increased level of an immune-response protein linked to inflammation. Those same women were also more likely to show signs of depression a year later.

Dr. Prather's study seems to suggest a complex feedback loop between a person's *physical* stress response and their emotions. This is one possible explanation for why people who aren't happy tend to have more health problems, while happier people tend to age better.

These studies echoed in my head as I talked to my husband's long-time internist, Elliot Aleskow, about what keeps Jim so young-looking and healthy. After Jim's last physical, Dr. Aleskow remarked that he would be out of business if everyone had an annual checkup like Jim's. But there's no chance of that; at his private practice in downtown Washington, D.C., Aleskow has spent 34 years treating a steady stream of stressed-out lawyers, lobbyists, and other professionals. Most of his male patients age 60-plus, he told me, are on two or three maintenance medications for, typically, high cholesterol, high blood pressure, and insomnia. "They can't sleep because of stress related to the job," he says.

Jim takes only one pill, Allegra, because he's allergic to our cat. That's it. So what makes him different? Honestly, Aleskow's answer surprised me.

"I think number one it's his positive outlook on life," he told me. "When he comes in, just his whole demeanor with others, he's just a happy person, and things feed into happiness. When you give him advice, he doesn't look at it negatively. He says, 'Oh, great, this is going to help, that's wonderful.'"

It's true that my husband has a general enthusiasm for life. Even if he has to work on the weekends, which he often does, he makes himself get up at 6 so he can get in and out of the office with enough time left in the afternoon to do something fun with us. When we go on vacation, he's usually the one pushing the rest of the family to get our bums off the beach and go exploring or hiking, which almost always ends up being more fun than what we were doing. Does all this mean he's happy? I decided to ask him (for the book, of course). I only slightly stood on his big toe.

"Are you happy?" I asked.

Long pause.

"Yeah, I think so," he said. I stepped off his toe.

Does this kind of verve for life make someone age better and live longer? Is it that such people are motivated to take care of themselves, as Dr. Aleskow sees in his practice? Is it the way such people handle stress? Or is it something no one has figured out yet?

Dr. Aleskow says happiness seems to impact your motivation to take care of yourself, live well, and stay healthy. "When someone has a positive outlook on life, they have a thirst for life, and when they have a thirst for life, they're motivated to do all those things that will make them healthier, age slower, and be in optimal condition," he says.

Conversely, people without a positive outlook often feel like life is a burden, and even more so when there's a health problem, which Aleskow sees regularly in his patients. "Someone like that might say, 'I'm having problems in my marriage, my kids are driving me crazy, and I just don't have the energy to really do anything. I'm at the point where I really don't care,'" he says.

> "My husband has a general enthusiasm for life. ... Does this kind of verve for life make someone age better?"

Aleskow's job seems to be part internist, part psychiatrist.

"That's most of what I do all day," he says. "How you interpret things that need to be done to better yourself, and to make the commitment to do that, is very important, ultimately."

Getting to Happy

What makes someone happy? That's a hard question to answer. When scientists try to gauge whether test subjects are happy, they don't ask it that way; they use scientific surveys that assess someone's emotional state in a variety of ways. After all, even generally happy people aren't always happy every minute (especially when someone's standing on their big toe).

But it's easy to look at someone like Jim and think he was just born that way. Indeed, all you have to do is look at a bunch of babies and toddlers to know that some people simply come into the world happier than others. But science suggests that's not the whole story—with Jim or anyone else. USCF's Prather explains that when it comes to happiness, "you have a genetic blueprint that sets certain parameters, and around those parameters there's room to wiggle."

So happiness is a lot like aging in general: your genes are the cards you are dealt, but if you play the game well, you can turn a poor hand into a winning game.

Scientists who study happiness have concluded that genetics accounts for about 50 percent of happiness. About 10 percent is attributable to circumstances. The rest, about 40 percent, is what you make it. Less-happy people can become happier, and even the happiest people can end up in an unhappy rut.

Jim experienced this, too, about 15 years ago, when his law firm hit a period of growth that placed a huge burden of additional work largely on Jim. Often working 7 days a week over a 2-year period, he had less energy, less desire to go out, a shorter temper, and he didn't sleep well. Photography, too, was an afterthought. We also fought more.

He became the classic stressed-out lawyer, the kind Dr. Aleskow sees all day long.

"What stress does is it just completely controls you to the point that you can't think or do anything else or care about anything else," Aleskow says. "What we *don't* do is we don't exercise when we're stressed, often, because we get so consumed by it. We don't eat right when we're stressed because we just want to grab something to squelch the stress, like a candy bar, which is a short-term antidepressant."

Eventually, this cycle takes its toll. "It's going to make you not look well, not feel well, not sleep well, and not have good relationships," he says. "You have to prioritize and say, 'I have to put my health, my looks, my feelings, first.'"

When Jim hired another lawyer to help handle the additional work, his stress began to ease, just enough to give him the impetus to start taking better care of himself. It was also around the time we had our first daughter, when he also began exercising regularly. It was just a little bit at first, even 5 or 10 minutes at a time, but whenever he did it, his mood lifted.

The biggest change in Jim's demeanor, energy, and happiness, though, came when he began improving his food choices. He kept saying he felt better, but it took about a year before I noticed what was right in front of me: he looked better, had more energy, and was consistently in a much better mood.

Jim didn't consciously make these lifestyle changes to become "happier." Mostly he just wanted to feel better. And he did end up feeling better, of course, but I think the greater benefit—to him and to his family—is that he was happier.

It turns out scientists have done a lot of research not only on what makes people depressed, they've also studied what makes people happy. The research isn't as robust because being happy is not a problem, and it doesn't have the same research urgency. But this research does offer some clues about what you can do, purposefully, to lift your enjoyment of life. Like anything else, it takes a little effort and training, but the brain is capable of learning a new approach to life just like any new skill. What's happening in the brain, explains Paul Nussbaum, the neuropsychologist, is "you're building up cellular connections where you don't have any." That's why it's hard in the beginning but gets easier with practice.

> "He did end up feeling better, of course, but I think the greater benefit—to him and to his family—is that he was happier."

So yes, some people are born with a better lineup of happiness genes— whatever that may be. But there are things you can do, according to scientists, to make yourself happier.

The Science of a Smile

A wide-ranging body of research exists about what makes people happy. Some scientists have found a link between *acting* happy and actually *feeling* happy. By making an effort to break the cycle of negative reactions and habits, it's possible to improve your level of happiness.

Charles Darwin was the first to suggest that smiling not only expresses our feelings of happiness, but actually makes us feel happier. On an MRI, smiling activates pleasure sensors in the brain, much like eating chocolate or winning money.

Frowning appears to have the opposite effect. A study out of Wales surveyed the emotional states of women who couldn't frown because of Botox injections. These women reported feeling happier than women who hadn't had Botox injections—but not for the reason you might think. The Botox women didn't report feeling any more attractive than the other group, which suggests that it was being unable to frown—physically—that kept their moods elevated.

Another group of researchers in Germany also looked at the impact of Botox on the connection between facial expressions and feelings. Scientists took MRI scans of subjects' brains while they made angry faces. Those who couldn't frown because of the Botox activated fewer areas of the brain involved in processing emotion than those who could frown.

There's a huge variation in how much we smile: research has shown that children smile the most—up to 400 times a day—but adults might smile anywhere from just a few times a day to about 20, or more. Not surprisingly, those who smile the least tend to be the least happy. That's why being around children often makes you feel happier: they smile a lot, and smiles are contagious. Maybe preschool teachers really do have it figured out!

But does it work to fake a smile even if you don't feel it? This area of research is less clear, but it does suggest that if you try to smile more often at moments in the day when smiling is appropriate—maybe if someone holds a door open for you, for example—it will have a reinforcing effect on your mood.

A smile gives you a fleeting mood lift, so the more you do it, the more it adds up to overall positive feelings, according to the research of smile expert Dr. Sonja Lyubomirsky of the University of California Riverside. The author of *The How of Happiness,* Dr. Lyubomirsky advocates being more aware of any upbeat emotions or reactions percolating inside you and letting them emerge as a smile. It will reinforce your positive feelings—and foment positive feelings in those around you, too.

Laughter works much the same way: scientists have shown that the act of laughing causes the brain to release endorphins, those feel-good hormones that enhance feelings of pleasure and dull feelings of pain. Happiness researchers like Lyubomirsky suggest that people figure out what makes them happy and then try to do more of that. Call it personalized happiness. So if you're feeling down, think about what makes you laugh and go do it. Maybe an evening of *Seinfeld* reruns will really help you face the next day.

> "A smile gives you a fleeting mood lift, so the more you do it, the more it adds up to overall positive feelings."

Things That Make You Happy

If you don't know what makes you happy, but you'd like to try to feel happier, science can still guide you. Research has found a few general principles of what will make you feel happier—or unhappier. These might be good places to start.

Social activity: The connection between social engagement and happiness has been shown in numerous studies. Being around others decreases negative thoughts, lowers stress, and boosts feel-good hormones in your brain.

But there's a caveat. People tend to adopt the ways of the people around them, both good and bad. So hanging out with a bunch of depressed people is not going to do you much good.

It may be difficult, but psychologists suggest taking a hard look at whether your friends are bringing you down, and if so, seeking other situations. Community activities such as church and volunteering might be good alternatives, and both are proven to be great mood-lifters.

Being in nature: Psychologists from the University of Rochester did a variety of studies to try to confirm the results of previous research showing that people feel "more alive" when they spend time in nature. These tests included leading college students on physically active 15-minute expeditions, both inside an office building and outside in nature. Students kept diaries of their activities and feelings while both indoors and out. Subjects were also asked to imagine themselves in various indoor and nature settings and report how they felt.

By every measure, the subjects felt greater vitality from being in nature compared with exploring an indoor environment. But strikingly, subjects reported similar positive feelings just from imagining themselves in nature.

Clock-Cheater Tip

Don't have time for a hike or can't get to the nearby park at lunchtime? Take a nature break at your desk by imagining yourself taking a peaceful walk through nature. Listen to birds chirping and brooks babbling, smell fresh grass and sweet flowers, touch soft moss and craggy bark, see rolling hills and colorful sunsets. Research has shown that this kind of exercise not only reduces stress, it also makes you feel happier.

Thinking rapidly: Have you ever had someone throw something to you while saying, "Think fast!" Next time it happens, your response should be, "Great idea!"

A team of psychologists from Princeton and Harvard were intrigued by the kind of fast thoughts people experience when they're manic, or excessively happy, such as after learning of a windfall or having a great new idea. They wondered if it worked both ways: if happiness triggers fast-paced thinking, can fast-paced thinking make you happy?

So the study asked test subjects to read different texts and statements, some with uplifting content and some with depressing content, both quickly and slowly. They also had them read the passages two different ways, rapidly and slowly. The study found that regardless of the content the subjects read, the

> "Regardless of the content the subjects read, the fast readers felt happier and had more energy."

fast readers felt happier and had more energy. In subsequent tests, a similar result was found by doing puzzles quickly versus slowly.

It's unclear why this worked, although it appears to be part of a deeply ingrained link in the brain between behavior and emotions. You can try it at home: next time you sit down to read try to speed up your reading tempo, or do an easy crossword you can speed through, and see how it makes you feel.

Things That *Won't* Make You Happy

Each one of us has specific people, places, or things that make us happy and unhappy. But scientists have found that some things appear to create, or reinforce, unhappy feelings.

Money: You've heard the saying, of course, and we know that money doesn't buy happiness. But scientists felt compelled to prove the point, and they did. Almost.

Research psychologist Dr. Ryan Howell of San Francisco State University asked 154 subjects to write a paragraph about a recent purchase and how they felt about it. Half wrote about buying an *experience,* such as going out to dinner, and half wrote about buying a *thing.* Those who bought an experience felt significantly happier about the purchase after the fact, leading Dr. Howell to suggest that having money only helps make you happier if it's used to buy experiences that create social engagement and good memories. (Of course, social activities that create positive memories don't have to cost anything!)

Researchers from Princeton, meanwhile, somewhat famously found that happiness does increase with income. But the effect only lasts up to about $75,000 a year in income—enough money to cover basic living expenses, health care, and some social experiences. Without having money for the things you really need, life can get pretty miserable pretty quickly, which is why the poor tend to be less happy. Anything over $75,000, though, seems to do little for your emotional well-being.

Watching TV: Researchers from the University of Maryland, College Park, studied 35 years of public opinion data from the General Social Survey, which not only tracks people's activities, but also asks for a self-reported measure of happiness. The approach has a little bit of a chicken-and-egg problem because it's not always clear if happy people do a particular activity frequently because they're happy, or if the activity itself is what's making them happy. But the data are still telling.

The list of activities surveyed covered a wide range, from the obviously enjoyable to the decidedly less so. The study included, among others, sex, sports, reading, cooking, paying bills, and home repairs. Surprisingly, watching TV was the only activity on the list "to correlate significantly lower with happiness," the authors wrote. They theorized that television, even though it's pleasurable, has no lasting happiness benefit and pushes aside other more mood-lifting activities.

Likewise, they wrote, television provides "a refuge for people who are already unhappy," such as people with poor social skills.

Multitasking: Sure, multitasking is bad in the boardroom or behind the wheel, but does it really make you less happy no matter when you do it?

Harvard psychologists Matthew Killingsworth and Daniel Gilbert had thousands of people report their activities and thoughts at random moments throughout the day, over several days, through an iPhone app. It's a tool called *experience sampling,* and in this case, it yielded fascinating results.

The pair found that nearly half of the subjects' thoughts through the day were not related to what they were actually doing. That may not seem like such a big deal; you probably do it, too. Who doesn't? But in this study, the subjects reported feeling the happiest when they were thinking only about what they were doing—even if they were doing something mundane. When

> "The subjects reported feeling the happiest when they were thinking only about what they were doing— even if they were doing something mundane."

analyzing the data, the researchers were able to conclude that "mind wandering in our sample was generally the cause, and not merely the consequence, of unhappiness."

There is a remedy, though, which is learning to be more mindful of what you're doing so you can live more in the moment—whatever that moment is. This kind of mindfulness is akin to meditation, and it takes a little effort and training, but it gets easier the more you do it.

Happy Trails

Psychologist Fred Luskin runs the Stanford Forgiveness Projects, a series of workshops and research projects at the university that investigate the impact of forgiveness. He also teaches a course on happiness at Stanford. If happiness can be taught, does that mean it can be learned?

It's more that people can learn to be happ*ier,* he says.

"Happier people spend a lot less time stressing about what needs to be changed in their life, and that is a huge relief to the mind and body," Dr. Luskin says. "And it's almost that simple."

Almost, but not quite. Happy people do a few other things, too, such as appreciate the people around them and feel grateful for small blessings, he says. To do that requires training yourself to see things differently and to make an effort to be happy, little by little.

Here are the things he tells his students to do to help them become happier people:

***Try* to be happy:** "If you have an intention of being happy, then you will pay attention to what makes you happy," he says.

Write your own happiness goals: Maybe it's having more friends. Maybe it's enjoying work more. Whatever happiness would mean to you, he says, picture it, ask yourself if you really want it, and decide if it matters enough to you to work at it. If so, start taking some tangible steps to get there.

Practice forgiveness: Luskin calls forgiveness a manifestation of happiness: you have to move past your resentments, or you can't maintain happiness. "[Resentment] blocks your vision of the goodness that's all over life," he says.

Will any of this make you age better? Happiness is such a personal feeling and can vary so much from day to day, moment to moment, that it's hard to view the pursuit of happiness and its impact on your health as anything but an intangible. But the science behind the role of happiness in longevity has become so much clearer, the effort is worth it.

Happiness researchers talk a lot about stress and the squelching effect it has on happiness. So for many people, just making a few better lifestyle choices, even small ones, will be enough to improve your quality of life just by reducing stress. But when combined with express efforts to be happier, the impact can be truly life changing. Nurtured over time, reduced levels of stress and greater feelings of happiness lead to better health and slower aging.

"It's hard to view the pursuit of happiness and its impact on your health as anything but an intangible. But ... the role of happiness in longevity has become so much clearer, the effort is worth it."

Looking Good, Feeling Good

As you've probably picked up on by now, remaining healthy and active throughout life will make you look and feel younger when you're older. A good diet, exercise, sleep, and well-managed stress can keep years off your face and body. The trick is establishing those habits early enough, and in a sensible way, so they stick and have time to make a difference.

But other aspects of aging—those often considered more cosmetic and less important to health—are, in fact, very important. A few purposeful changes can help stave off some of the other not-so-welcome characteristics of aging, such as wrinkles, tooth decay, hearing loss, and vision loss.

It's not vanity; it's humanity.

Having more wrinkles than you think you should, for example, can affect the way you feel about yourself. Gum disease, a common ailment in the elderly, can make you sick—literally. But it's a manageable condition. Losing your hearing in your 70s or 80s can be very isolating, and it becomes hard to stay connected to the life you know. Yet being socially connected is a key component of preventing cognitive decline. If you develop vision problems, you'll end up living with the constant frustration of not being able to drive or read, which can lead to clinical depression.

Who spends time envisioning a future with wrinkles, dentures, hearing loss, and low vision? Few people worry about these aspects of growing old because they certainly don't seem to be health problems on par with getting Alzheimer's or losing the ability to walk—the kinds of age-related ailments many people *do* worry about. But these are concerns that should be right up there with keeping your brain, your heart, and your muscles healthy. They are, in fact, central to your future quality of life.

Saving Your Skin

Ask any dermatologist about the best way to prevent skin aging, and the answer will be instantaneous: avoid sun damage. But we're not getting the message.

The American Academy of Dermatology conducted an online survey of adults age 18 and older, released in May 2012, about spending time in the sun and tanning. The study proved that cultural messages die hard, even in the face of irrefutable scientific evidence. In this case, the American ideal of beauty still includes a tan, even though it's been proven and publicized that sun exposure causes wrinkles and skin cancer.

> "The American ideal of beauty still includes a tan, even though it's been proven and publicized that sun exposure causes wrinkles and skin cancer."

According to the study, 58 percent of adults 18 to 29 thought people looked better with a tan and 71 percent thought that sun exposure was "good" for your health.

This helps explain, at least in part, why Medicare claims for treatment of nonmelanoma skin cancers doubled between 1994 and 2006.

Of course, the sun does have important health-promoting properties and shouldn't be shunned. The body uses sunshine to make vitamin D, an important nutrient essential for the body to absorb calcium, making it critical to bone health. Vitamin D also has been shown in studies to help protect people from various kinds of cancer (ironically), autoimmune diseases, and high blood pressure. (See the later "Ageless Advice" chapter for more guidance about getting enough vitamin D from the sun; it varies enormously based on your skin type and where you live.) Sunshine also means being outside, which is good for exercise and stress reduction.

But without the right understanding of the risks and rewards sunshine offers, people often don't take the time to protect their skin from the powerful age-inducing effects of the sun. They will stay out in the sun, unprotected, knowing they're likely to get a sunburn—much the way they might decide to eat an ice cream even when they're trying to lose weight. It's a classic example of the present self being unable to relate to, and worry about, the experiences and feelings of the future self.

But understanding the science behind a sunburn will help you appreciate the long-term damage it can cause. When you stay in the sun too long and your skin turns red, there's a lot going on inside your skin cells.

Ultraviolet (UV) light from the sun is an extremely strong form of energy, and when it passes through your skin, it hits water molecules inside your cells. This energy causes some of the oxygen molecules in that water to lose an electron and become free radicals. When a radical bounces around inside a cell, it damages anything in its path in a desperate attempt to find a second electron to bind to so it can become stable again. With prolonged sun exposure, this constant exposure to UV light means a tremendous number of radicals are zooming around inside your cells, damaging them from the inside.

Your body does the best it can to defend itself. It marshals its antioxidant resources to squelch as many radicals as it can. Some research suggests people with diets high in antioxidants are better able to fight off these kinds of assaults—another reason a diet high in fruits and vegetables is good for your skin. But when antioxidants can't keep up with the havoc wreaked by free radicals, your immune system is mobilized to start repairing the damage. That immune response causes inflammation, just as it does when your body tries to repair the damage from a twisted ankle or a bruise. When it happens inside your skin cells, your skin becomes visibly red, swollen, and painful. That's a sunburn.

Over time, sun damage like this accumulates in your cells. Every time your body repairs cell damage from a sunburn, the impact appears to go away. But with repeated cycles of damage, your cells can't recover to their original state, much the way a cracked wall is never quite the same after it's been repaired. It may look just as good for a while, but cracks will gradually appear where the repairs were made. The same is true for your skin cells: the more sun exposure they get, the weaker they are from the constant cycle of damage and repair. In the end, they lose structure and elasticity, which shows up on your skin as wrinkles—or worse.

"There's a chain reaction that occurs and leads to damage," explains Tom Slaga, pharmacologist at the University of Texas Health Science Center in San Antonio and an expert on skin cancer. "Too much of it, and the damage builds up and eventually you get cancer or you have aging of the skin. Your skin thins anyway with age, so to add a lot of sunlight on top of it, that's where you end up with the most damage."

Tan Damage

A tan is part of the body's defense system. Your skin cells release pigment to help absorb UV light and prevent cellular damage from free radicals, causing it to turn brown. A tan may look attractive, but it's another sign of cell stress. That's why people who spend their lives getting tan in the sun or tanning salons, even if they don't burn, get wrinkles earlier and have a higher risk of skin cancer.

The best way to take care of your skin, then, is to protect it from sun damage and nourish it from the inside. Eating a good diet full of vitamins, minerals, and antioxidants gives your body better resources to limit damage to your skin cells so they stay healthy and young-looking.

Beyond that, there's no big secret to preventing skin aging, says dermatologist Dr. David Green of Bethesda, Maryland. "In terms of priorities, environmental injury trumps everything—all the lotions, potions, and exfoliation you can do, can't undo the bad things we do," he says.

Cleansing and moisturizing are basic hygiene everyone should do to keep their skin clean and moist, but that won't prevent wrinkles, Green explains. "Most wrinkling is not the result of dry skin," he says. "There are people who have very oily skin who have a lot of wrinkles."

Dr. Green points out that if you take a person with any type of skin and any level of wrinkling on their face and then look at the skin on their buttocks, which generally gets no exposure to sunlight, you'll see dramatically less wrinkling. Point taken.

For people who already have some wrinkling they'd like to deal with, dermatologists and other skin experts tend to agree that lotions with alpha-hydroxy acid, vitamin C, and other antioxidants—and even old stand-by creams like Retin-A—can help minimize the appearance of age lines. Other experts suggest trying to reduce squinting (using glasses for vision or sunglasses for outdoors), which can prevent deep wrinkles around the eyes. And sleeping on your back can keep wrinkles from getting creased into your cheeks and mouth when you sleep.

My husband, who has astonishingly youthful skin, has done none of that; he has had the same basic skin-care routine for 40 years. He washes his face with warm water and Neutrogena soap and then splashes his face with the coldest water he can get out of the tap. He moisturizes every morning with basic Olay face lotion, which he thinks he might have originally borrowed from a girlfriend in college—and he's still using it!

> "If you take a person with any type of skin and any level of wrinkling on their face and then look at the skin on their buttocks ... you'll see dramatically less wrinkling."

However, Jim is very careful about getting too much sun. He has olive skin to begin with, and people with more pigment in their skin are less prone to sun damage because that pigment absorbs more of the ultraviolet light. But even though Jim is naturally more protected than I am, with my fair skin, he still uses sunscreen on his face, especially whenever he's going to be out in the sun for more than 15 minutes or so.

What's been most dramatic, though, is how little Jim's skin has aged since he started eating so many whole grains and antioxidant-rich foods. In fact, more than just not developing any new wrinkles, his skin is smoother and brighter than it used to be. It's obvious he's protecting his skin from the inside out.

Teeth for All Time

Good dental hygiene is not only good for your teeth and smile, it's also good for your health. Scientific literature is brimming with studies that link poor oral health to a host of chronic and acute diseases, including these:

- Cardiovascular disease
- Diabetes
- Poor pregnancy outcomes
- Respiratory disease
- Osteoporosis
- Cancer

The link stems from gum disease, often called periodontal disease or gingivitis. This chronic oral health condition comes from long-term exposure of the gums to plaque on the teeth. Plaque is a sticky film on the teeth made of food particles, mucus, and bacteria. If plaque isn't effectively cleaned from the teeth by good brushing and flossing, it can turn into tartar, a harder deposit that tends to collect around the gumline. The problem is that plaque and tartar irritate the gums, which can initiate a cascade of systemic responses.

Dentist and registered dietitian Charlene B. Krejci of Case Western Reserve University recently reviewed the scientific studies that have looked specifically at the link between oral health and women's health. Published in the journal *Oral Health and Preventive Dentistry* in 2012, her review explained that plaque and tartar release "toxic products" that cause the gums to get inflamed, leading to mouth ulcers, tissue deterioration, bone and tooth loss, and inflammation throughout the body.

"An increased concentration of circulating inflammatory markers has been directly correlated with the presence of the disease," Dr. Krejci wrote. In study after study, gum disease has been closely linked with the presence of inflammation throughout the body. Systemic inflammation is associated with a wide variety of chronic health conditions and diseases.

So it's clear that once you get advanced gum disease, you're doing the rest of your body no good. Scientists still haven't pinned down the exact role of inflammation in disease, but it's generally believed that controlling inflammation is an important part of staying healthy as you age.

Oral health studies have not necessarily been able to conclude specific cause and effect: does poor dental hygiene cause systemic disease, or is some behavioral or environmental trigger causing both? More likely, researchers believe, there's a cycle involved, with health factors such as smoking, obesity, and low socioeconomic status leading to multiple health problems, including dental disease. People with little money often have less access to good dental care and may not have the educational programs that teach them how to take care of their teeth. When dental disease sets in, it exacerbates other conditions that may be present as a result of poor lifestyle habits.

> "Plaque and tartar release 'toxic products' that cause the gums to get inflamed, leading to mouth ulcers, tissue deterioration, bone and tooth loss, and inflammation throughout the body."

The message is clear: don't put off going to the dentist, at least once a year, and every 6 months is recommended. Cleaning your teeth is not just about cleaning your teeth: the effect of regular dental hygiene adds up to a healthier mouth as you age, which contributes to better health overall.

Hear the Future

My father lived a long and healthy life until his recent death at age 89. He was a historian and an intellectual interested in every aspect of culture, from music to architecture to literature. He was not an athlete, but throughout his later years, he religiously took long walks around the neighborhood. In bad weather, he would drive to the airport just minutes from Washington to walk the distance of the terminal several times. Yet this man who didn't smoke, wasn't overweight, and exercised regularly could do nothing about the hearing loss that plagued him in the last 15 years of life and the vision loss that made his last 5 years frustrating and, at times, outright depressing.

When my father's hearing began to go, it became hard for him to converse in noisy situations. Then it became difficult to follow the conversation even among his wife and daughters, although one could argue whether he wanted to, of course! Eventually, his hearing trouble made it nearly impossible for him to carry on a conversation unless the acoustic conditions were perfect. It also robbed him of the great pleasure he derived from classical music. We intervened with whatever amplification devices we could, but it didn't do enough.

My father's experience made me determined, personally, to do whatever I can to prevent the same kind of a sensory loss he experienced. Luckily, the best time to start such prevention tactics is midlife, although it's never too late.

Hearing loss typically begins in your 40s, even if you don't notice it. Much of the current scientific knowledge about age-related hearing loss focuses on cumulative exposure to noise. That's a really important point. Some noise exposure is just unavoidable—it's a noisy world. But if you reduce your exposure to loud noise wherever you can, you are eliminating one level of cumulative damage and protecting your hearing in the long run.

> "Hearing loss typically begins in your 40s, even if you don't notice it."

Try, for example, turning down the volume to a level you can just comfortably hear—whether it's the television, the radio, or through headphones. If you really like to listen to loud music, try to do it less often.

Also use hearing protection. Earplugs are a great way to deal with loud noise. Buy a pack of disposable foam plugs or reusable earplugs, and use them whenever operating loud machinery, hunting, or during any other high noise exposure. I've just started using earplugs when I use a hairdryer every morning (and I've discovered that not all earplugs are created equal, so it takes a little testing with different types and brands). According to the CDC, hair dryers have the same noise-level rating as a power lawn mower!

Hearing loss has also been linked to oxidative stress, and recent research has been focused on possible supplements that may help prevent such oxidative damage from leading to hearing loss. Unlike many other cells in the body that can be replaced when oxidative stress leads to cell death, cells involved in hearing do not regenerate. So high levels of oxidative stress can lead to irreversible hearing loss.

A great deal of research currently focuses on the potential impact certain vitamins, minerals, and antioxidants can have on preventing hearing loss. A study published in 2011 by researchers at the University of Sydney in Australia found in a 5-year study that people with the highest vitamin A levels in their blood had a 47 percent decreased risk of hearing loss, while those with high dietary intake of vitamin E had a 14 percent reduced risk of hearing loss.

Other studies have found protective effects from various nutrients, especially antioxidants, suggesting that acute free-radical damage occurs after exposure to loud noises, and antioxidants can help repair that damage. Studies have shown better recovery after loud noise exposure using high doses of antioxidants and other micronutrients, including these:

- Vitamins E and C
- Alpha lipoic acid, an enzyme found in meat, fish, chicken, and other foods

- Glutathione, an antioxidant found in many foods, including cruciferous vegetables such as broccoli and cauliflower
- Magnesium, found in dark green leafy vegetables

This research is still developing—some has only been done in rats and guinea pigs—so it's hard to say yet which supplements will clearly help prevent hearing loss. But the evidence suggests that protecting your hearing is yet another reason to eat a healthy diet with plenty of fruits and vegetables, providing at least the minimum recommended intake of vitamins and minerals.

But like the advice to limit your sun exposure to best protect your skin, most hearing experts still say noise reduction will make the biggest difference in preventing hearing loss for the average person. So before you crank up the music, think of the last time you had a conversation with someone who was hard of hearing, and picture yourself in that person's position. It may give you just enough motivation to keep the volume a little lower. Over time, that may preserve your ability to listen to music at all.

See the Future

An ophthalmologist recently told me that even though I have no vision problems (other than needing drugstore reading glasses), I should start getting annual ophthalmologic exams when I turn 50. Why? Because both my father and my maternal grandmother suffered from macular degeneration in their 80s, so my family history puts me at risk in the future. And of course, I fully intend to be living that long (I also fully expect my husband will be cranking along right with me!). So this warning hit home.

Macular degeneration is a condition in which the center of the retina, or the macula, gradually deteriorates. It is one of the most common causes of vision loss in people over age 65; about a third of adults age 75 and older have some degree of the disease.

Macular degeneration gradually caused my father to lose the ability to comfortably read the newspaper, magazines, and books. Combined with his hearing loss, it intensified his feelings of isolation, and at times it made him feel pretty low.

According to the American Health Assistance Foundation, the biggest risk factor for macular degeneration is age, but there are others:

- Family history
- Smoking, which restricts blood flow, causes damage to the retina because it's a big consumer of oxygen
- Oxidative stress, which is thought to worsen the progression of macular degeneration
- Obesity, characterized by a body mass index greater than 30, which can more than double the risk of getting macular degeneration
- A high-fat diet or nutrient-poor diet, especially one low in antioxidants, which is another known risk factor
- High blood pressure, which also restricts blood flow, reducing oxygen to the retina
- Lack of exercise, which can keep blood and oxygen from flowing adequately throughout the body, and also to the eye and the retina
- Prolonged exposure to the sun, which can allow ultraviolet radiation to get into the eyes and cause deterioration of the retina (People with light-colored eyes seem to be at greater risk, perhaps because their eyes have less pigment to absorb the UV rays.)

Two large studies have evaluated the effectiveness of dietary supplements on eye health and on macular degeneration in particular.

The first Age-Related Eye Disease Study (AREDS) found that high levels of certain antioxidants, along with zinc, significantly reduced the progression of macular degeneration. The supplements tested included the antioxidant vitamins E and C along with beta-carotene. These micronutrients don't appear to prevent the onset of macular degeneration, but they may keep it from worsening.

A follow-up study that began in 2006, called AREDS2, is testing the same supplements as the original study, but with the addition of omega-3 fatty acids and the antioxidant lutein. Results are expected in 2013.

The science suggests that both vision and hearing loss can be prevented to some degree by staying healthy and active, but especially by eating a diet high in vitamins and antioxidants. Unlike hearing loss, though, which can also be prevented to a large degree by reducing exposure to loud noise, vision loss is harder to prevent by taking any single precaution besides optimizing your general health.

Part 7

Action Plan for Aging Less

Making It Happen

This book is full of reasons why making a few key changes to your lifestyle can help you live a longer, healthier life. For some people, these changes may seem pretty big. But I hope the clearest message in this book is that these changes can be made slowly, in small increments, and over time, so they're easy and will become lasting habits.

The science is clear that slow and steady progress toward a healthier lifestyle can pay huge rewards as you age. My husband's experience has borne out the effectiveness of that approach and shows that transforming your life does not have to be a wrenching, painful experience. But the more you know about what you're doing, the easier and less painful it will be.

Can you really make big changes in small doses? The answer is a resounding "*Yes!*" In fact, for most people, that's the only way to do it.

Changing your routines and habits is hard. Many people *try* to adopt new behaviors, or ditch old ones, yet success stories are relatively hard to come by. The nation's weight problem is probably the best example. Although glossy magazine covers tout the 30- and 60-pound weight-loss stories of stars like Kelly Clarkson and Beyoncé Knowles, for every person you know who has lost 10 pounds in the past year, you probably know five who have gained that much. If it were easy, celebrity weight-loss "strategies" wouldn't be cover-story fodder.

Most people don't have cooks, nutritionists, trainers, and a cover-story photo shoot to keep them on track, so how can the average person make lifestyle changes that will both make a difference and stick? Whether it's weight loss, eating more nutritious food, exercising more, reducing stress, or sleeping more, the first step is understanding the science so you know exactly how the changes you make affect your body—right down to your cells.

You can't see yourself aging day to day, week to week, or even month to month (as hard as you might look). The changes your body undergoes as time passes are so incremental they're virtually invisible—until they build up enough that you can see them. Even if you wish you couldn't.

And therein lies the biggest challenge when it comes to engaging in habits that will slow down the aging process. If you can't see yourself age, you certainly aren't going to be able to see yourself aging *less*. At least, not for a while. So how do you know if it's working?

Aging more slowly is not like losing weight, which you can watch happen by the numbers on a scale. To change the way you age, you have to *know* that what you're doing is making a difference. You have to *know* that the antioxidants in the blueberries you just ate are helping your body neutralize the radicals causing damage inside your cells; that taking a brisk walk is making immune cells flow out of your bone marrow to boost your resistance and your muscles are generating new mitochondria; that turning off the TV and going out with your friends, even though you're tired, is helping your brain preserve connections—and perhaps build new neurons; and that staying up too late will make you eat more the next day and reduce your resistance to colds.

> "If you can't see yourself age, you certainly aren't going to be able to see yourself aging *less*. ... So how do you know if it's working?"

If you've read this far, you've taken the first step already: learning about the underlying science of aging (or the most important points). So now that you know more about how it works, and how your daily decisions affect the aging process, all you need is a system to implement those changes in a way that's doable. You have two choices: exerting your willpower and changing your habits.

Jim has approached his change in lifestyle primarily as an adjustment to his habits, done with minimal exertion of willpower because the changes he made along the way were so incremental. There's a lot to be said for this approach, even if it takes a little longer to get to your goal. And there will always be times when you need your willpower to follow through.

So you need both techniques, but they'll work best if you understand how and why they work.

Waking Your Willpower

If you've tried, and failed, to eat less, exercise more, control your spending, save money, go to sleep earlier, stop procrastinating, spend less time online, or anything else you knew you really *should* do, you've probably chalked it up to lack of willpower. Along with that, most likely, came a sense of failure because people naturally equate willpower with strength, resolve, and accomplishment. So when you can't summon enough willpower to do something you know you should do, you feel weak, powerless, and ashamed.

But you shouldn't, for a variety of reasons. It's better to understand your willpower—because you do have it, even if you don't know how to use it effectively. Based on that insight, you can try different approaches that will likely be much more successful.

Willpower is challenging for a variety of reasons, one of which is that our brains aren't wired to resist many of the temptations we face. The kinds of things people tend to indulge in, such as excess calories and sweets, exert such a strong pull on us because they were necessary throughout evolution. The prehistoric parts of our brain want us to eat as much as we can whenever food is plentiful. Sweets, in particular, represent a dose of concentrated, easily accessible energy that was useful for survival throughout evolution. The human brain is wired to compel us to accumulate excess energy when it's available. That's why eating something sweet makes us feel so good: it was an evolutionary

> "Understand your willpower—because you do have it, even if you don't know how to use it effectively."

adaptation that encouraged us to eat foods that provided such a concentrated dose of calories.

Willpower, meanwhile, comes from our ability to plan for the future and control ourselves. It is the ability to *not* do something in order to gain a future benefit. But this skill came later in human evolution; throughout its existence, the human species' biggest concern has always been short-term survival because humans didn't live into old age until very recently. So your brain isn't always good at imagining the future in a meaningful way. That only makes it harder to exert the willpower you need to make difficult decisions today that will help you in the future.

Many studies demonstrate this. Hal E. Hershfield, PhD, research psychologist at New York University, for example, looks at how this plays out in the way people save for retirement. In one study, he asked adult subjects to think about themselves and about other people, both currently and in the future, while undergoing an MRI. In some subjects, the same region of the brain was activated when thinking about themselves currently and when thinking about themselves in the future. But this was not true of everyone. Some people, when thinking about their future selves, used parts of the brain typically used to think about *other* people. For these participants, thinking of their future selves was like thinking of someone else.

Why does this matter? Dr. Hershfield asked the study subjects to do a test in which they planned how much money to save for the future. It turned out that those who thought of themselves in the future as someone else were the ones who saved the least.

It's not an impossible problem to overcome. In a related experiment, Dr. Hershfield asked college students to make theoretical decisions about long-term savings and investments. But before making their financial decisions, some students were shown photographs of themselves that had been age-progressed by special software. Seeing pictures of themselves decades older made the subjects feel more connected and sympathetic to their future selves, and in response, they "allocated more than twice as much money to the retirement account," the study says, as the subjects who did not see the pictures.

Jerry Seinfeld touched on this aspect of human nature in a way anyone can relate to in a standup routine about staying up too late and not getting enough sleep. The comedian said that when he stays up too late, that's a decision made by Night Guy. Night Guy doesn't have to worry about not getting enough sleep because that's Morning Guy's problem. Poor Morning Guy is powerless. He has to get up after just 5 hours of sleep, and all he can do is curse Night Guy.

But it's more than fodder for a funny routine. Someone who doesn't feel connected to his or her future self is more likely to make the kinds of choices that have long-term negative consequences—such as spending too much, getting too much sun, and overeating. Most people don't have access to age-progression software (although there are programs online that will do it for a fee), but if you're someone who tends to make decisions that are bad for your future self, you can try a couple exercises to help make the future you seem more real.

Start by spending time with any older people you know, even your own parents, and when you're with them, really pay attention to what their lives are like. Notice what's different about how they live, and try to picture yourself with the same living circumstances or ailments. How would you like your life to be the same or different?

Or just take a minute or two every day to envision your future life, all the way down to the minor details, such as how mobile and healthy you are, based on what you can expect given your current life habits.

These exercises don't have to be depressing; they're simply a way to train your brain to make a stronger connection between your present self and your future self. Not all brains make that connection very strongly. It's a mental exercise like mindfulness or meditation that will get easier over time so that eventually you'll have a better

> "Someone who doesn't feel connected to his or her future self is more likely to make the kinds of choices that have long-term negative consequences—such as spending too much, getting too much sun, and overeating."

connection between your current and future selves, which should help you make better long-term decisions.

The Willpower Way

Other problems with willpower may be easier to overcome. The next time your willpower wanes, look at what you had done in the previous 12 or 24 hours. Did you get enough sleep? Did you eat badly? Did you have a fight with your husband, wife, or co-worker? Had you already resisted temptation multiple times?

Scientists have found that all these things can interfere with your ability to exert optimal willpower. Often what feels like a personal failure is really an environmental one. The solution, therefore, is to optimize your environment.

> "Your desires come from a different spot in the brain than your sense of self-control .... One part says, *I want to eat that brownie,* while the other part says, *I shouldn't eat that brownie.*"

Because your desires come from a different spot in the brain than your sense of self-control, when you feel a battle waging inside your head, it's because a battle really *is* waging inside your brain. You may well be getting powerful signals from different parts of your brain to do opposing things. One part says, *I want to eat that brownie,* while the other part says, *I shouldn't eat that brownie.*

But scientists are learning that just as the brain can be trained to learn new tasks, the part of your brain you want to *win* these willpower battles can be strengthened so it can fight back more effectively. Willpower isn't a muscle, but scientists are learning that it behaves a lot like one. Studies have shown that willpower ...

- Uses tremendous energy.
- Can be strengthened over time.
- Can suffer from overuse.
- Will rebound after resting.

- Is restored after eating.
- Doesn't work well when you're tired.
- Is highly susceptible to stress and illness.

Dr. Kelly McGonigal, research psychologist and lecturer at Stanford University and author of *The Willpower Instinct,* explains that you have to understand willpower, and how it works, to use it most effectively. Always pay attention to the situation when your willpower fails you. Were you tired? Hungry? Was it late at night? These are common problem areas when willpower often fails. Here are her suggestions:

Get more sleep: Studies have shown that willpower falls off dramatically when you get less than 6 hours of sleep, so it's the equivalent to being a little drunk. "When you don't have enough sleep, your brain has a hard time using energy efficiently," she says. "The energy-costly acts of the brain become impaired first—the prefrontal cortex, which is responsible for controlling impulses, focusing on tasks, and remembering your long-term goals."

Start early: If you have to take on a big willpower challenge, try to do it earlier in the day. Willpower is "like a battery that's recharged by sleep" and drains throughout the day, she says.

Give up the guilt: If you fail at doing something you wanted to do, just accept it. Rather than beat yourself up for that one failure, focus on the reasons your willpower sagged and try to fix those reasons, such as getting more sleep. Guilt over failing is one of the main factors why people fail even more spectacularly. This so-called "what the hell effect" is why people who blow their diet on a bowl of ice cream might give in and eat the whole pint. But McGonigal says a single setback here and there should not be a big deal. "Single setbacks are not predictive of long-term success, as long as you don't let it slide into multiple days of doing it," she says.

> "Guilt over failing is one of the main factors why people fail even more spectacularly."

Don't drain your brain: Exerting self-control, McGonigal says, takes more energy than anything else the brain does. So if your brain is already managing a high level of stress, your chances of having strong willpower are much lower. Take stress-reducing steps like going outdoors, spending time with animals, meditating, deep breathing, sleeping, prayer, yoga, or other diverting or relaxing behaviors. "Anything you do that reduces stress helps your brain use energy more efficiently," she says.

Allow a reward: The human brain likes a reward, which is why people love gambling and lotteries. So when you need to do something hard, engage the motivational side of your brain by giving yourself a reward after you've done the tough task. Maybe you can plan to have a coffee break after you've written a full page. Or let yourself buy a new lipstick after you've exercised. It's not cheating because you still have to want to succeed to make it work. But giving yourself a reward will "capitalize on every kind of motivation you have," McGonigal says.

Notice the short-term benefits: If you're trying to establish a new habit that will have long-term benefits, it can be hard to stay motivated. McGonigal suggests also focusing on the short-term value, such as an opportunity to spend time with a friend or daily time to just take care of yourself. "Find the daily payoff," she says.

Psychologist Roy F. Baumeister has found that willpower is more effective shortly after an infusion of glucose—which is what food turns into after it's broken down and reaches the brain. Your brain is a huge energy consumer; it only weighs about 3 pounds, but it uses about 25 percent of all the glucose you get from your food. And the brain works better when it's well fed. A trip to the grocery store is good enough proof for me: if I'm hungry when I shop, I end up buying all kinds of things I don't need but that seemed like a good idea at the time. So this research suggests you should avoid making tough decisions with long-term consequences unless you've eaten recently.

Dr. Baumeister's work on willpower, recently adapted into the book *Willpower* with journalist John Tierney of *The New York Times,* also explains that willpower can be trained like a muscle—at least to a point. But it can be strengthened a lot more than most people think, using many of the tactics outlined in this chapter, especially paying attention to the interaction of eating patterns and decision-making.

Watching Jim transform his diet and lifestyle has taught me that establishing good habits is every bit as important as willpower—and probably easier, as long as you do it right.

I know what you're thinking: you'd have lots of good habits if only you had the willpower. But if you change your habits slowly, a tiny bit at a time, you won't need as much willpower as you might think. As Jim has developed his habits, it's been easier for him to exercise willpower.

Tiny Habits

A tiny movement has grown into a mini-revolution online in the past year: it's called Tiny Habits. It's the brainchild of experimental psychologist and consultant B. J. Fogg, PhD, who runs the Persuasive Technology Lab at Stanford, focusing on creating behavior change and habits. Some of Fogg's students at Stanford have gone on to make millions of dollars in technology ventures, in part by utilizing the kinds of techniques they learned in his classes about how to change the consumer's behavior. The founders of Instagram were his students, for example, among others.

Late in 2011, Dr. Fogg decided to try a personal experiment, outside his teaching at the university or consulting for high-tech clients. He set up a small, free, email-based service to help people change their habits, which he named 3 Tiny Habits. It was based on everything he has learned about what makes people change from studying human behavior over 18 years. On his website, he explains that "when you know how to create tiny habits, you can change your life forever."

Fogg's basic premise is that "if you are using willpower to change your habits, you will probably fail." Instead, his approach is that whatever you want to change has to be *tiny*—as in, virtually insignificant. For example, a Tiny Habit, by Dr. Fogg's measure, is flossing one tooth or doing one push-up. A habit is only tiny, he says, if it takes almost no effort, it's virtually painless, and it takes 30 seconds or less.

People who register for the weekly program read the rules and then have to list the three Tiny Habits they plan to do that week. Each day that week, Fogg sends out an email the participants have to answer.

The hardest part has been getting people to follow the rules, Dr. Fogg says—that is, getting them to pick a tiny-enough habit. "One of the things I say is, 'imagine willpower doesn't exist and then describe what you want to do,'" he says. "Every Tiny Habit should take almost no effort. Don't do twelve push-ups, do one. What you're trying to develop is not the ability to do push-ups. You already know how to do push-ups. What you don't know is how to do it *automatically,* and that's what you have to focus on. It's about the automaticity."

If you do 12 push-ups, he explains, your brain won't want to do it again because the experience will be unpleasant. Maybe not very unpleasant, but unpleasant enough that it will take some willpower to make yourself do it every day. But under Fogg's program, all you're interested in at the outset is ensuring you always do your Tiny Habit, so you want to make it willpower-free and easy as pie. Once the habit is there, you can do anything with it, and it will take far less effort.

> "Fogg's basic premise is that 'if you are using willpower to change your habits, you will probably fail.' Instead, his approach is that whatever you want to change has to be *tiny.*"

The ultimate goal is to turn a new habit into an "anchor" habit, like brushing your teeth or taking a shower. An anchor habit is one you keep doing, with no prompting, guilt, or extra thought, even if you miss a day because something in life went haywire (and it always will). It has to be routine.

Dr. Fogg's online program took off immediately, and within 6 months, several hundred people were signing up each week. The program has had a "phenomenal" success rate, Fogg says. But successful at what, exactly? Doing one push-up? Yes and no.

A large portion of Fogg's Tiny Habit participants follow through on their Tiny Habits for the week. But in their emails, including follow-ups weeks or months later, they also have been telling Fogg how much their habits have expanded beyond the Tiny level. One man, for example, emailed he was doing 500 push-ups a day, "and he started with one," Fogg says. He is thrilled to have been a catalyst for this man's success, but not surprised. Once you've created a habit, Fogg explains, it naturally grows: flossing one tooth for a week naturally grows into flossing two or three teeth, and then your whole mouth, because the act of flossing becomes routine.

Habits grow on their own for two reasons, Fogg says. First, the more you do something, the easier it gets and the less motivation and willpower it takes to do it, so you naturally do more. And second, succeeding at a Tiny Habit provides almost immediate positive reinforcement: people feel proud of themselves for making a positive change in their lives, and it spills over into other areas.

"When they succeed on these tiny things, they get so excited and they're like, 'oh my gosh, I've actually succeeded on this.' They get energized to take on big things," Fogg says. "There seems to be this feeling of, 'I'm awesome, I've gotten in control of this aspect of my life.'"

Dr. Fogg does not advise taking on one Tiny Habit at a time, but rather making several at once. And he suggests breaking down your habits into two types: those that need to grow, and those that don't. Always putting your car keys on the hook by the door is a habit that doesn't need to grow. So is always telling the waiter at a restaurant you don't want any bread and butter brought to your table. This is Fogg's special (easy) trick to keep him from eating bread and butter with dinner. It's far easier to tell the waiter not to bring it than to summon the willpower to resist it after it's arrived!

A habit you want to grow is different and may require a little knowledge. When the goal is a big one, like losing weight, he says, it's helpful to learn more about the subject before they can break it down into baby steps. The most important part, Dr. Fogg says, is choosing the right small step: it has to be appropriate, scalable, and of course, tiny.

Habits in Our House

Jim has been living the Tiny Habits routine since long before Tiny Habits existed. Maybe not exactly—he never did just one push-up at a time, for example, but he has lived this program in spirit. It's the approach that ended up changing his entire approach to health, fitness, and aging.

By taking the smallest steps aimed at getting more fit, more healthy, and more balanced, Jim has gradually become dramatically more fit, more healthy, and more balanced than he was 10 years ago. Would it have been better if he had made all the changes he's made over the past 10 years all at once when he was 54? I doubt he would've been able to stick with them, and even if he had, he might never have stopped "missing" his old ways or feeling constantly deprived. But the way it unfolded, the new Jim not only doesn't miss the old Jim; he feels more nourished and more fulfilled than ever.

Jim talks about habits now like they're easy to acquire. In fact, I'd have to say he's devoted to his good habits and is constantly on the lookout for new ones he can adopt. Success at adopting better habits has made it easier to take on the challenge of adopting new ones. Now he enjoys trying something new—and he's doing it all the time—because he's figured out that if you start small and let it grow organically over time, it doesn't have to be stressful.

> "By taking the smallest steps aimed at getting more fit, more healthy, and more balanced, Jim has gradually become dramatically more fit, more healthy, and more balanced than he was 10 years ago."

You may remember that when Jim started exercising regularly, he began with just 10 minutes a day, or sometimes less. My reaction at the time was, *Really? Ten minutes?* But that 10 minutes grew to 12. And then 15. And then 18, and after a year, it was 20 minutes. Now it's 30 to 40 minutes at least every other day and only on rare occasions does he feel the need to force himself to do it (when life has been especially tiring, usually). Exercise, for him, has become routine.

The Tiny Habits concept is perfectly suited to the goal of better, slower aging. A Tiny Habit may take more time to turn into something meaningful than making a big change through sheer willpower—even if you have a better understanding of willpower. But aging takes time, so when it comes to getting your habits right, you have some time to work with.

The drawback of making small changes is that you may not notice the benefit right away. But the psychological lift of continuing the habit anyway—which you can do because it's small and painless—may be enough to keep you going because you know you're making a difference. Knowing that the science backs up what you're doing makes any change more meaningful. Tackling those changes one small step at a time makes doing it more possible.

Ageless Advice

If I could break down this book into three essential points, they would be this:

- Changes to improve your health and fitness are easy to make if you start small enough.
- These changes can dramatically slow down the aging process if you stick with them over time.
- Understanding the science behind how these small changes are benefitting you will help you stick with it until the effect is obvious on the outside, too.

All the information you need to put those points to work is in this book, but sometimes it helps to have a step-by-step action plan. After all, there's no substitute for direct advice.

What follows is some of the specific guidance I have garnered from hundreds of scientific sources and experts, combined with my firsthand knowledge of what has worked for Jim through his successful transformation. He began as a regular guy with an average diet and average physical fitness and became a regular guy with a superior diet and excellent physical fitness. Along the way, he acquired a better outlook, more energy, and a younger-looking appearance. You can, too.

As I've said before, if you've read this far, you've already taken the first important step to aging less and living longer, which is learning about the physical effects of certain behaviors. So what you'll find in this chapter are habits you can tackle in various areas that will make a big difference to your health over time, with some suggestions of ways to get there.

Talk to Your Doctor

The tips in this chapter are aimed at the typical healthy person, so if you have any medical issues, please talk to your doctor before taking on any new lifestyle or diet changes.

Start at the beginning of the list or at multiple places at once. But pick just one or two changes to start—and go for ones you *know* you can stick with. When you're comfortable with those changes, add another one or two, even if it's a few months later. Don't be limited by what's written here. For example, where I say eat an apple as a midday snack every day, B. J. Fogg would say eat just one *bite* of one apple every day. He would also say pick more habits at once, but make them smaller.

Whatever approach may suit you, start by figuring out the level of change you can commit to, however small it is, and start aging less. And as Stanford psychologist Kelly McGonigal points out, the effort you make to change your habits or lifestyle is in itself "protective." Just *trying* to age better helps you age better.

Notch Up Your Nutrition

Add one fresh vegetable to one meal, once a day. Cook and treat your vegetable as little as possible, so try a dark green salad, lightly steamed broccoli, or green beans boiled just until tender. Frozen vegetables are okay, too, but don't overcook them or add butter, salt, or cream sauce. A small portion is fine, but work your way up to having at least one fresh or lightly cooked vegetable at lunch and dinner every day. Then start eating larger portions of vegetables by cutting back on other items on your plate. Vary what you eat, too, so you get lots of different vitamins and minerals.

Pick a fruit you like, and eat it once a day. Maybe throw an apple in your bag every morning before work and eat it for a midmorning snack. Or cut up half a melon and keep the chunks in the fridge so it's always there to grab and eat. Start with a regular time to eat your fruit—such as after lunch or work. Aim for fruit with a lot of color, such as berries, red grapes, watermelon, cantaloupe, or kiwi. Frozen is fine, but you shouldn't add any sugar, so fresh might taste better.

Eat smaller portions. You don't need more than 3 ounces protein in a meal. Try using smaller plates, and use colored plates that match the color of your food. Cut back just a tiny bit so you hardly notice the difference. Then cut back some more.

Try more nonanimal protein sources, such as black beans, nuts, and tofu. There's a reason why so many people in the world love these foods: they may be out of the ordinary for you, but they are delicious and very good for you. Millions of people can't be wrong.

Switch to leaner portions of red meat. Trim what you eat so you don't eat a lot of fat.

Avoid processed meats, such a hot dogs, bacon, and bologna.

Let yourself get really hungry before you eat. Try to stretch out the length of time between meals. Even try fasting one day or evening a week.

Add more gently cooked foods to your diet to reduce your consumption of advanced glycation end-products (AGEs). Look for opportunities to bake, poach, or stew your food instead of frying, broiling, or grilling it. If it doesn't make a difference to you, go for gentle, slower, lower-temperature cooking.

Reduce Your AGEs
AGEs, or advanced glycation end-products, are toxic compounds that form when food or meat is cooked with such intense heat that it browns, caramelizes, or chars. AGEs also form under intense dry heat, so a lot of processed foods have high AGE contents, too. They taste good, but when overconsumed, AGEs can contribute to a host of health problems, including diabetes, heart disease, and cancer.

Switch from refined to whole grains. Look for opportunities to replace white bread, rice, and pasta with whole-wheat bread, brown rice, and whole-wheat pasta. Soft-style whole-wheat breads can make the switch easier. At first, do it just once a day—maybe for your toast at breakfast. Try different types of whole-grain products, and when you find one you like, start using whole wheat all the time. This change can take a while! With rice and pasta, also do it gradually; try mixing together regular and whole-grain versions at first so you get used to the change in flavor.

Cook with healthy oils, such as olive, canola, or grapeseed oil instead of butter.

Eat healthy snacks and treats. Instead of junk food or unhealthy, fattening desserts, start looking for healthier treats you like. Satisfy your sweet tooth—especially between meals—with a granola bar, yogurt cup, or oatmeal cookie. Try to enjoy the process of finding (or baking) something you like!

Cut back on sugar. Reduce the sugar amounts in recipes and look for sugar on food labels. Use sugar substitutes sparingly, if possible. They aren't good for you either, and a good goal is gradually getting used to having a less-sweet diet. It doesn't have to be painful!

A Low Goal

New sugar-consumption guidelines from the American Heart Association recommend no more than 5 teaspoons a day for women—that's 20 grams—and 9 teaspoons a day for men—that's 36 grams. For children, it's 12 grams, or 3 teaspoons. Treat that as a goal, and cut back gradually.

Eat more slowly. This helps you enjoy your food more and keeps you from eating so much. This technique alone will make you more mindful about what you eat.

Start counting calories, or at least notice them. Some foods are much higher in calories than you think. If you know a frozen coffee drink has 800 calories (a whole meal's worth!), will you still want it?

Drink alcohol in moderation. Try to limit yourself to about one drink a day, especially wine. Cut back gradually.

Get a physical. Talk to your doctor about your goal to age better. If you're worried about your diet, ask if you can have your vitamin and mineral levels checked so you know where you need to improve.

Eat some omega-3 fatty acids every day, through your food or a supplement.

Take a multivitamin every day.

Weigh yourself. If you hate to do this, start by getting on the scale every day without looking at your weight, just to get in the habit of stepping on the scale. The process of standing on the scale repeatedly will make it less anxiety-provoking. Then, when you feel better because of other changes you've made, you can start looking at your weight. By then, it'll be a habit.

Exercise, Exercise, Exercise

Take a walk! Five minutes, ten minutes, once around the block—it doesn't matter what you do, just plan to do it every day or almost every day. You can also use the treadmill, exercise bike, or elliptical machine. Just figure out what you can manage based on your time and schedule, and get started. Move briskly, but stop before you get uncomfortable. If you're just able to carry on a conversation while you exercise, but not too easily, you're at the right intensity level. If you can't stick to the amount of exercise you started with, cut back and try again. Wait until you *want* to do more before you start adding more time. You'll know it when you feel it. And remember, build up slowly. Your ultimate goal should be 20 minutes of brisk exercise seven times a week, 30 minutes four or five times a week, or 45 minutes three times a week. It could take weeks, a year, or even longer to get there. It took Jim 3 or 4 years to get to his schedule of 30 to 40 minutes four times a week, but now it's easy for him.

If you miss a day, don't stress about it. You're not preparing for a marathon, you're trying to establish a new habit.

Do some strengthening exercises, such as push-ups (even if you start with just one!), sit-ups, or free-weight exercises. Try alternating your walking and exercising days, and eventually work up to doing strengthening work every time you walk (or run or bike).

Don't Overdo It!

When you start exercising, it's easy to do too much at first. You may not feel like it's too much while you're working out, but you will feel it later. And then it's too late because your brain won't want to do it again. Until exercise has become an ingrained habit you know you'll keep doing, keep it at a pleasurable level so you'll want to do it again. Eventually, pushing yourself hard will feel good, and you'll still want to go back for more.

Exercise with a buddy or group of friends. Or form a support group that emails every day about what exercise you did. That extra social support is motivating and fun.

Boost Your Brain

Read something every day. Whether it's a book, a magazine, or a newspaper, reading helps keep your neurons intact.

Learn more. If there's a subject that interests you, find out more about it. You'll build new connections in your brain that will help protect you from cognitive decline later.

Socialize. Interacting with people is one of the best ways to keep your mind agile and your gray matter active. If you're not crazy about your friends, find new ones through a hobby, church, or community program.

Make a skills list. On the right side of a piece of paper, write some things you're good at. On the left side, write some things you aren't good at. Then pick something from the left side and start doing it. It will be uncomfortable and maybe not that enjoyable at first. But that's to be expected, and it's part of the reason to do it. You're training your brain to make new connections, which you want to do to keep your brain healthy. Once those connections are there, that skill will feel easier and more pleasurable. Calligraphy, anyone?

Find something meaningful to you, whether it's a hobby or volunteering. Having a sense of purpose in life, especially if you share it with others, protects your brain. And it's fun.

Manage Stress

Sleep more. Try to go to bed a half an hour earlier than usual, and don't work right before bed. Aim for at least 7 hours a night as a goal. Move your bedtime up 15 minutes at a time, or less, stopping for a month or two with each advance. If you normally go to bed at 11:30, for the next month, go to bed at 11:20.

Practice mindfulness, or living more in the moment. Make yourself focus on what you're doing, even if it's something mundane. It takes effort, but it *will* get easier.

Take a meditation or yoga class. Practice at home. Even better, practice with a friend. Don't worry if you feel like you're bad at it. With time, you'll get better, and just the process of learning to meditate helps your brain stay young.

Do deep-breathing exercises. Deep breathing slows you down and reduces your stress. This simple technique is a great way to make a difference when you need a quick way to calm your mind and reset patterns of negative thinking.

Get out in nature. Listen to music. Play with an animal. Take a warm bath or hot shower. These are all relaxing and help relieve the chronic effect of stress.

Hug and cuddle your spouse and kids more. Tender touching releases hormones that relieve stress.

Find reasons to smile and laugh. Watch some standup comedy if that works for you. Whatever it takes, get some of those happy-feeling facial expressions in your life every day because they reduce stress.

Sleep More

Learn to value sleep. Start noticing the difference in the way you feel, behave, and work after a good night's sleep. It's critical to your health, so try to appreciate it. This attitude change is necessary for many people who take sleep for granted!

Establish a sleep-focused bedtime routine, such as reading in bed before you fall asleep. Try not to do any email or computer time right before going to sleep. If you're sleepy during the day, that's a signal you need more sleep.

Try a mini-meditation moment if you wake up during the night. Lie still and listen to your breathing while trying to push aside all your other thoughts. It will be very hard at first, but just like training a muscle, it will get easier and more effective. So don't give up if it doesn't work at first.

Have Better Sex

Talk to your doctor if you have sex problems. If your doctor doesn't know about your issue, he or she can't help. People in relationships with good sex lives are happier, are more satisfied emotionally, and stay together longer.

Cuddle, hug, and touch more. These stimulating activities release many of the same pleasure and bonding hormones as actual sex and draw a couple closer together, which leads to more and better sex.

Have a sex talk with your spouse or partner. Set up a time to talk when you can both be unemotional and straightforward. Talk about what you like and don't like. Don't be offended, and try to avoid being offensive.

Aim to have sex at least once a week. Some studies suggest having sex twice a week, if you're in a relationship, yields the best health and emotional benefits.

Boost Your Happiness

Decide to improve your happiness. Think about what makes you happy, and try to do more of it. It can be small: if contacting old friends would make you happy, write a letter to an old friend. Happiness does not have to be nebulous—you can take concrete steps to be happier.

Find things to do that make you smile and laugh. These actions alone make you happier, and when you're happier, you'll do them more, creating a positive cycle of better feelings.

Evaluate your friends. Are they making you unhappy? If so, try to socialize more with other friends who make you feel happier.

Spend more time in nature. Take regular hikes or nature tours. Anything that gets you into semi-wilderness will lift your spirits. Also try walking on grass in your bare feet whenever you have the chance.

Imagine yourself in nature. If you can't get out, take a nature walk in your mind! Smell it, hear it, and feel it all around you. In some studies, this exercise is almost as mood-lifting as an actual walk outside.

Make yourself think faster. Push yourself to read and do puzzles faster than normal. It's an exercise that lifts your mood.

Have Fun with Your Hobby

Rekindle an old hobby, find a new one, or love your current one. If you've had a hobby in the past, start it up again. If you don't, think about what you'd enjoy doing. Enjoy experimenting while you look! Hobbies have a huge health payoff as you age.

Take a class that interests you at your local community center.

Volunteer. This is a hobby that helps you age well and benefits others at the same time.

Help your child start a hobby. You can be the hobby helper, and you might get interested yourself.

Beef Up Your Body Care

Use sunscreen anytime you'll be in the sun for prolonged periods.

Keep a sunscreen stick or small tube in your car, purse, or other bag so you don't accidentally get caught in the sun for more than 15 minutes. Fair-skinned people should spend less time outside unprotected than darker-skinned individuals, and people farther north can spend more time outside before getting burned than those close to the equator. Don't allow your skin to turn more than the barest touch of pink before covering up or applying sunscreen.

> ### Clock-Cheater Tip
> Depending on your skin type, expose your face and arms, or arms and legs, to the sun for 10 to 20 minutes three times a week in warm weather months so your body makes enough vitamin D. If you do this regularly during the spring, summer, and fall, your body will have stored enough vitamin D to last all winter.

Use a moisturizer that contains sunscreen.

Brush your teeth twice a day, for at least 1 minute each time.

Floss your teeth daily. You can always start with one tooth at a time!

Go to the dentist twice a year, or at least once a year, to get your teeth cleaned.

Wear sunglasses to prevent squinting (to prevent wrinkles) and UV damage to your retinas (to protect your vision).

Turn down the volume of your music, especially if you listen through headphones or earbuds.

Use ear protection if you're exposed to loud noises regularly, even the hairdryer.

And finally, don't rush! Pick the ideas in this chapter that appeal to you the most and seem manageable, but break them down in whatever way works for you. You can refer to the list again in a month or two for more inspiration. But for now, don't think about how incorporating these activities into your routines will change your life. Think of it as changing the way you age. In time, that *will* change your life.

Fabulous Foods

So many foods have been studied for their health benefits, but the results tend to dribble in and get buried in the rest of the day's news. In this appendix, I share some of Jim's favorite foods—which we eat a lot of—that also have been shown, in recent studies, to have great health benefits. Most of these foods not only have lots of vitamins and minerals, but are also high in antioxidants and fiber.

This small list is by no means complete, but it includes some fruits, vegetables, grains, and nuts that are generally easy to find in supermarkets, even if many people don't necessarily regard them as superfoods or regularly consume them. This list is a great place to start as you try to boost the nutritional content of your diet by adding new and cell-friendly foods. Use this list for inspiration to step out of your comfort zone and try something new that will do your body good!

A little later, I provide some cooking tips and a few recipes that are some of my family's favorite healthy dishes made of really good-for-you ingredients.

Notable Nutrition

The U.S. government recommends eating a wide range of fruits and vegetables, and one way to do that is to eat a variety of colors. That's generally a good approach because different colors often indicate the presence of different micronutrients. But sometimes it's also good to just know what vitamin you're getting. If reading this book has made you more determined to get plenty of vitamin E in your diet, for example, you need to know which foods are a good source of vitamin E.

Now Serving ...

The government defines a fruit or vegetable "serving" as about ½ cup or 1 average-size piece of fruit and recommends 5 to 13 servings a day, depending on how many calories you eat. That's a lot, but don't be put off. Even if you can't eat that much, you should still eat whatever you can in the way of fresh fruit or vegetables (and nuts and grains). The vitamins, minerals, and antioxidants in these foods are going to help your health no matter how much you eat, so even one is better than none. Once you establish the habit, you can build up over time!

Here are some of the particular health benefits that have been identified for a few favorite foods, along with any notable micronutrient content. Just about everything on this list is rich in natural, plant-based antioxidants of one kind or another, and many are high in fiber.

Whole Grains

Grains are plant-based foods just like fruits and vegetables, so they contain many of the same healthful components. Unlike refined grains, whole grains include the super-nutritious bran and germ of the original plant, which hold most of the nutrition. In addition to varying amounts of vitamins and minerals, whole grains provide fiber and natural phytochemicals, which can have powerful antioxidant and anti-inflammatory properties. Even one serving a day can make a significant difference to your health if consumed over many years!

Brown rice: Thanks to its high fiber and antioxidant content, compared with white rice, studies have shown brown rice reduces the risk of diabetes, enhances weight loss, and can reduce the risk of some cancers. *Notable nutrition:* magnesium and manganese.

Oatmeal: In human and animal studies, the soluble fiber in oatmeal has been shown to help protect against atherosclerosis, lower cholesterol, improve cardiac health, and reduce the risk of breast cancer, among other benefits. *Notable nutrition:* phosphorus, magnesium, and selenium.

Popcorn: Popcorn contains polyphenols such as ferulic acid, an antioxidant and anti-inflammatory polyphenol. If you cook your popcorn in oil or smother it with butter and tons of salt, you'll cancel out popcorn's healthful properties, so make it air popped with just a little sprinkle of salt. *Notable nutrition:* fiber and polyphenols.

Whole-rye bread: Compared to whole wheat, animal and human studies have shown whole-grain rye can help reduce body weight, improve insulin response, keep you full longer, reduce inflammation, and better control the expression of some risky genes. *Notable nutrition:* manganese, B vitamins, and selenium.

Whole-wheat flour: Whole-wheat products are now commonplace, making eating whole grains easier. People whose diets include grains that are primarily 100 percent whole grains, such as whole-wheat bread and pasta, have been shown in many studies to weigh less and have a lower risk of diabetes, asthma, cardiovascular disease, heart disease, and cancer. *Notable nutrition:* manganese and magnesium.

Clock-Cheater Tip

Some people are turned off by the taste of whole-wheat flour, which is nuttier and richer than white flour. If you're one of those people, look for whole-wheat pastry flour at your local health food or gourmet supermarket. Pastry flour is ground finer than regular whole-wheat flour and, therefore, has a more subtle, tender texture. It's virtually unnoticeable in cookies, cakes, pastries, and even pancakes, especially if you mix it with a little bit of white flour. It's a great way to make your favorite treats more nutritious!

Vegetables

Vegetables come in so many types, there's something for everyone. But the best way to eat them is to go for as wide a variety of colors as possible to get a good mix of vitamins, minerals, and phytochemicals. Also, generally the nutritional value of vegetables is best preserved when they're not cooked very much, although there are some notable exceptions, such as tomatoes, which have a higher level of the antioxidant lycopene if they're cooked. Try not to use unhealthy fats, cream sauces, and lots of salt, although a sprinkle of salt and pepper can do wonders for some vegetables!

Bell peppers: These vegetables contain a range of beneficial antioxidants that have been shown to contain anticancer and anti-inflammatory properties, including age-related brain inflammation, in animal studies. *Notable nutrition:* vitamins C and B_6.

Broccoli: Studies have shown broccoli contains sulforaphane, a potent antioxidant that can suppress the expression of genes that play a role in cancer and heart disease. It has also been shown to reduce inflammation and improve gut health. Raw or lightly cooked broccoli is best. *Notable nutrition:* vitamins K, C, and A and potassium.

Cabbage: A cruciferous vegetable like broccoli, all different types of cabbage have been shown to have potent anticancer properties, thanks to high levels of antioxidants and other phytochemicals. It's highly anti-inflammatory, benefits digestion, and helps cholesterol levels, in part because of its high fiber content. It's most beneficial when lightly cooked. *Notable nutrition:* vitamins K and C and folate.

Green, leafy vegetables: Among the most nutrient-dense foods on the planet, greens contain high levels of potent antioxidants and many vitamins and minerals. They're linked to a reduced risk of cancer, Alzheimer's disease, heart disease, and more. Choices include Swiss chard, romaine lettuce, kale, spinach, and mustard greens. *Notable nutrition:* great for hard-to-get vitamin E and iron, among many others.

Sweet potatoes: This nutrition powerhouse is packed with more antioxidants, vitamins, minerals, and fiber than any other vegetable, ounce for ounce. Some of the world's healthiest people eat large quantities of sweet potatoes. These tubers are best consumed with a small amount of healthy fat to maximize nutrition absorption. *Notable nutrition:* vitamins A and C, beta-carotene, and potassium, just to name a few.

Nuts and Legumes

With their high protein content, vitamins, and wide range of anti-oxidant phytochemicals, nuts and legumes are a great way to spruce up your diet. Just $1/4$ cup nuts is a great snack that packs lots of nutrition and can really blunt your hunger. Legumes are a nutrition-packed staple throughout the world and make a great substitute for meat once in a while.

What's in a Name?

Peanuts aren't actually nuts. They're legumes!

Almonds: These nuts are linked to lower "bad" LDL cholesterol, reduced risk of heart disease, and better blood-sugar regulation. *Notable nutrition:* vitamin E, potassium, and protein.

Beans: High in protein, fiber, minerals, and antioxidants, but low in fat and sugar, beans have great health benefits. Studies have linked them to reduced risk of heart disease, cancer, obesity, and diabetes, and to greater longevity. *Notable nutrition:* iron, zinc, folate, and calcium.

Edamame: These fresh soybeans, often eaten cooked as a snack food, are loaded with protein, fiber, and antioxidants but low in fat. They have been linked to lower inflammation and better blood-sugar regulation. *Notable nutrition:* vitamin C, folate, and manganese.

Pistachios: Packed with antioxidants, these nuts have anti-inflammatory properties and have been linked to lower "bad" LDL cholesterol and lower risk of cardiovascular disease. *Notable nutrition:* thiamin, vitamin B_6, manganese, and copper.

Walnuts: Packed with more antioxidants than any other nut, as well as healthy fats and a healthy form of vitamin E, walnuts are linked to lower weight gain, better cardiovascular health, reduced inflammation, and lower risk of cancer and diabetes and cognitive decline. *Notable nutrition:* omega-3 fatty acids, manganese, copper, and protein.

Fruit

In general, fruit contains high levels of vitamins, fiber, and anti-oxidants, which makes almost all fruit good for you. But some fruits have been identified in scientific studies as having particularly good health benefits, and those are the ones I've included here. And the whole fruit is always better than the juice, which may have sugar added and some or all of its antioxidant capacity and fiber stripped away.

Apples: Apples have been linked to a longer lifespan in lab animals; lower "bad" LDL cholesterol levels in human studies; and reduced risk of various cancers, infections, and Alzheimer's disease. *Notable nutrition:* vitamin C.

Berries: The antioxidant levels in berries are hard to match in any other food, and they're high in fiber, too. They have been linked to lower rates of cognitive decline and better memory, lower "bad" LDL cholesterol levels, better cardiovascular health, reduced risk of cancer, and stronger bones. *Notable nutrition:* vitamin C, calcium, potassium, and folate (depending on type of berry).

Grapes, red: Another kind of berry, red grapes contain a huge array of antioxidants. Garnering the most attention is resveratrol, a potent antioxidant that recently has been found to have antiaging properties by stimulating genes that affect longevity. Resveratrol is also linked to a reduced risk of diabetes and obesity. Red grapes have been linked to better blood-sugar regulation, cardiovascular health, and cognitive function. Moderate consumption of red wine, made with red grapes, draws its notable health benefits from this remarkable fruit. White grapes are nutritious, too, but they don't have the same level of bio-active compounds as red grapes. *Notable nutrition:* vitamins C and K.

Kiwi: For a fruit, kiwi has an extremely broad range of nutrients, as well as essential amino acids involved in fighting cancer and preventing heart disease. Kiwis contain more vitamin C than an orange the same size. Kiwis have been linked to less DNA damage from oxidative stress, reduced risk of blood clots, and better cardiovascular health. *Notable nutrition:* vitamin E, potassium, copper, vitamin C, vitamin K.

Prunes: This underappreciated dried fruit (really a dried plum) has enormous health benefits—far beyond the "regularity" you probably already know about. They are among the best treatments available for increasing bone density and can actually reverse bone loss. Their unique and powerful combination of antioxidants is especially good at preventing free radical damage to fatty tissues, including cell membranes and the brain, and provides many other health benefits. Prunes also contain soluble and insoluble fiber and many vitamins. *Notable nutrition:* vitamins A and K.

Watermelon: This humble picnic fruit is high in vitamins and fiber, has few calories, and contains the well-studied antioxidants beta-carotene and lycopene, which have been linked to a reduced risk of asthma, cancer, and heart disease. More impressive are studies that show watermelon's high concentration of two particular amino acids, l-citrulline and l-arginine, can lower blood pressure and improve cardiovascular health. *Notable nutrition:* vitamins C and A.

Other Foods Jim Regularly Eats

And to round out the list, here are some more foods Jim often snacks on.

Chocolate, dark: This sweet treat contains high levels of antioxidants that help the body increase production of nitric oxide, which can improve blood pressure and cardiovascular health. Dark chocolate has been linked to reduced risk of heart disease and stroke. *Notable nutrition:* flavonoid antioxidants.

Tea: With high levels of antioxidants, tea has been linked to many health benefits, including lower risks of cancer and cardiovascular disease. Green tea, in particular, has been found to be beneficial in part because it contains sulforaphane, the same powerful phytochemical in broccoli. But some studies have found no health benefits, so more research is needed. *Notable nutrition:* polyphenol antioxidants.

Yogurt: This fermented dairy product provides great protein and other major health benefits. In studies, the regular consumption of yogurt has been linked to greater longevity, increased immune response, lower "bad" LDL cholesterol, higher "good" HDL cholesterol, lower body fat, denser bones, lower risk of cancer, and even fresher breath. Look for yogurt with live cultures, less fat, and low sugar content. *Notable nutrition:* iodine, calcium, phosphorus, and zinc.

A Few Family Favorites

It's easy to eat more fruit, but many people don't know much about how to cook vegetables so they turn out both healthy and delicious. Find a vegetable-focused cookbook for reference. (I use *The Victory Garden Cookbook* by Marian Morash.)

Here are a few of my family's favorite preparations and cooking techniques, to help you get started eating more healthful, age-defying vegetables in your diet. They are super easy for a weeknight meal, too.

Steamed Broccoli

Forget the special steamer basket—you don't need it. Put $1/2$ inch water in the bottom of a 2-quart pot, cover, and bring to a boil over medium heat. Add a little salt to the water if you'd like (as we do).

Add 2 cups chopped broccoli florets and stems, not cut too small. (Each piece should be about a mouthful.) Cover and cook for about 2 minutes or until water returns to a boil. Reduce heat to low, and cook for 3 more minutes or so. Without opening the lid, remove from heat and leave covered for 5 more minutes. The broccoli should be bright green and just tender. Drain and serve.

To make it more flavorful and add a dose of healthy omega-3 fatty acids, toss your broccoli with 1 tablespoon extra-virgin olive oil, a hefty squeeze of fresh lemon juice, and salt.

Variation: If you've never much liked broccoli, try this: steam as directed, but use chicken stock instead of water. Even broccoli haters will like it prepared this way!

Sautéed Cabbage

Thinly slice $1/4$ to $1/2$ head regular cabbage, and break it up so it falls into thick shreds. In a large frying pan over medium-high heat, heat 1 tablespoon canola or other light-tasting healthy oil, such as safflower oil. Add the shredded cabbage and toss for 2 minutes.

Add $1/4$ cup chicken stock or water and 1 teaspoon salt, reduce heat to medium, cover, and cook for 5 or 6 minutes, tossing every minute or so, until cabbage is just tender. Season with salt and fresh ground black pepper.

Brussels Sprouts

These delicious, incredibly healthy vegetables often get a bad rep—mostly because they're usually cooked badly and taste bitter as a result. Try this instead:

Trim the stems off the brussels sprouts, and cut the sprouts into quarters. You should have about 2 cups. Bring 2 quarts water to a boil, and add 1 teaspoon salt and the brussels sprouts. When the water returns to a boil, cook for 2 or 3 more minutes. Sprouts should be bright green and tender. Drain and toss with a pinch or two of fresh-grated lemon zest (lemon juice makes them lose their appealing bright-green color), and a drizzle of light olive oil or a small pat of salted butter.

Sweet Potatoes

Pick sweet potatoes that are relatively even in shape (so they cook evenly) and heavy for their size. Preheat the oven to 400°F. Prick the sweet potatoes a few times with the point of a knife, and place them on a piece of aluminum foil (this is important) directly on the oven rack. Bake for 30 to 45 minutes, depending on the size. When they're done, a sharp knife should glide in easily into the center of the sweet potato. Let cool for 5 minutes, slice open, and sprinkle with fresh lime juice and salt.

You can also peel and slice sweet potatoes and steam the chunks, or scoop out the flesh of the baked sweet potato and mix with a little light olive oil and salt into a rough mash.

Salad Dressing

Use this healthier alternative to creamy or store-bought dressing. Using a fork or a whisk, combine 3 tablespoons extra-virgin olive oil, 1 tablespoon wine vinegar, fruit vinegar, balsamic vinegar, or another good-quality vinegar, salt, and pepper.

Use this dressing on leftover vegetables such as broccoli, green beans, asparagus, cauliflower, cabbage, cooked or raw carrots, or a mixture of any of these to make a quick and healthy vegetable salad for lunch or dinner on a hot day.

Variation: For a sophisticated dressing, add ¹/₂ teaspoon Dijon mustard. For a flavorful dressing, include 1 or 2 pinches chopped garlic or shallots. For an aromatic dressing, stir in 1 teaspoon chopped fresh herbs such as dill or basil. For a sweeter dressing, add 1 teaspoon fresh squeezed orange juice in place of 1 teaspoon vinegar.

Quick Chicken Salad

You'll need 1 large chicken breast, poached, or use the breast from a rotisserie chicken. Shred chicken into a bowl. Add ¹/₄ cup light mayonnaise, ¹/₄ cup light sour cream or plain Greek yogurt, ¹/₄ cup coarsely chopped walnuts, ¹/₄ cup coarsely chopped celery, and ¹/₄ cup tart, crisp apple, skin on, cut into ¹/₂-inch cubes. Mix thoroughly, and season with salt and pepper.

Baked Lemon Chicken Breasts

Preheat the oven to 400°F. In a baking dish, combine 2 teaspoons butter and 2 tablespoons extra-virgin olive oil, and place in the oven until butter is melted and just starting to bubble.

Meanwhile, as butter melts, cut 2 large boneless, skinless chicken breasts into 4 equal pieces, and arrange them on a large piece of waxed paper or plastic wrap with plenty of room between pieces. Cover with another layer of waxed paper or plastic wrap. Using a meat pounder or the back of a heavy pan, pound the breasts until about ¹/₄ inch thick. Remove the top layer of plastic wrap, and squeeze the juice of ¹/₂ lemon over the breasts and season with salt and fresh ground black pepper. Using a fork, turn over each piece of chicken. Drizzle with juice from the other ¹/₂ lemon, and lightly season with a little more salt and pepper.

Remove the baking dish from the oven, and using a fork, pick up each breast, quickly place it in the butter–olive oil mixture, turn it over, and leave in the dish. Repeat for each piece of chicken, coating both sides in the butter and oil. Arrange pieces so they're as close to one layer as possible, cover dish loosely with aluminum foil, and return to the oven. Bake for 15 minutes. Serve each person 2 pieces of chicken and a few spoonfuls of sauce. Try it with brown rice and plain steamed broccoli.

A Final Touch

A great time to add a piece of fruit to your day, or even just a few cut pieces of fruit, is right after lunch or dinner. It cleanses the palate, gives your meal a refreshing finishing touch, reduces your craving for dessert, and gives you one more serving of fruit.

Learn More, Live More

This book breaks down the process of aging into its basic mechanisms so you can understand what your body is going through and appreciate the impact even small changes in your lifestyle can have on your health and longevity, especially when you let them build up over time. I've aimed to make this information easy to grasp and not overwhelming, with the hope that it will encourage you to start small, with purposeful, but not painful, choices that will improve your health for years to come.

But a lot more information is available from many wonderful sources, so I encourage you to keep looking and learning. The more you know, the easier it is to make the right decisions to help you look younger and feel better at any age. Information is inspiration.

To help get you started, here are a few smartphone apps and online resources for guidance and information on all aspects of health and aging—many of which dovetail with the advice in the book. Use these to expand your knowledge; help establish new habits; and start living a better, longer, younger life!

Smartphone Apps

EatChewRest
Do you eat too fast? If so, this app sets a time to chew and a time to just stop and appreciate your bounty. It's good for hitting the reset button if you'd like to try eating slower and more mindfully.

Go! To Sleep
This app from the Cleveland Clinic helps evaluate your sleep habits and quality so you can make pointed changes to get more shut eye.

MyFitnessPal
Whether or not weight loss is one of your goals, it's a good idea to know how many calories you're eating. This is a great on-the-go database for most mobile systems, covering calorie counts for 1.5 million foods.

Nap26
Suzanne Somers' nap app uses specially orchestrated rhythms and relaxing music to lull you into the perfect 26-minute nap and wakes you when you feel rested and relaxed. Even if you don't sleep, it's great stress-suppressing break from the daily grind.

RunKeeper
Keep track of your new walking (or running or biking) program with your smartphone's GPS function. Use it to set goals (remember to start small!), track your progress, get a little extra coaching, and even create a workout soundtrack.

Websites

American Federation for Aging Research
afar.org/infoaging
This site contains the latest research on aging and is very easy to navigate.

ChooseMyPlate.gov
myplate.gov
The U.S. Department of Agriculture's main consumer nutrition website is extremely thorough, with information broken down by age, food groups, interest level, and profession.

Micronutrient Research Center

lpi.oregonstate.edu/infocenter

The Linus Pauling Institute at Oregon State University is one of the leading research centers on vitamins, minerals, and antioxidants, and its web-based Micronutrient Research Center has extensive information about scientific research and findings related to nutrition, health, and aging clearly laid out.

National Institute on Aging

nia.nih.gov

The official website of the National Institute on Aging also has excellent consumer advice and information on every aspect of aging, all very simply explained.

The Nutrition Source

hsph.harvard.edu/nutritionsource

The Harvard School of Public Health has an excellent website with clearly written, scientifically based information on many aspects of nutrition and health.

RealAge

realage.com

This website by celebrity doctors Michael Roizin and Mehmet Oz is not only informative, but fun, too. It has a little bit of a supermarket-magazine feel (as in, "6 Shocking Truths About Eye Health"), but the information is sound, often fascinating, and presented in easy-to-consume nuggets. Plus, taking the RealAge test to find out how old you really are is enough to get you hooked—on the website and on taking better care of yourself.

Science*Daily*

sciencedaily.com

This online magazine is a great resource for the latest research on topics related to health and aging, among other scientific topics.

SELF Magazine NutritionData

Nutritiondata.self.com

This is an astonishingly comprehensive nutrition database for thousands of food items, including whole foods and commercial items. It's just really interesting to look through, although sometimes a little distressing, such as when finding a favorite food that isn't so favorable.

3 Tiny Habits

Tinyhabits.com

This weekly program was developed by experimental psychologist B. J. Fogg, director of Stanford University's Persuasive Technology Lab. An expert in getting people to change their behavior, Fogg's online program encourages people to make tiny—and he means really, really *tiny*—changes to their habits weekly. When you register, you get Fogg's complete rules, which you must follow exactly, he says, or it won't work. You'll get encouraging missives through the week.

Index

··· Q–R ···

···· S ····